T0249732

Gender Affirmation Surgery in Otolaryngology

Editors

REGINA RODMAN
C. MICHAEL HABEN

OTOLARYNGOLOGIC CLINICS OF NORTH AMERICA

www.oto.theclinics.com

Consulting Editor
SUJANA S. CHANDRASEKHAR

August 2022 • Volume 55 • Number 4

ELSEVIER

1600 John F. Kennedy Boulevard • Suite 1800 • Philadelphia, Pennsylvania, 19103-2899

http://www.oto.theclinics.com

OTOLARYNGOLOGIC CLINICS OF NORTH AMERICA Volume 55, Number 4
August 2022 ISSN 0030-6665, ISBN-13: 978-0-323-96173-8

Editor: Stacy Eastman
Developmental Editor: Diana Grace Ang

© **2022 Elsevier Inc. All rights reserved.**

This periodical and the individual contributions contained in it are protected under copyright by Elsevier, and the following terms and conditions apply to their use:

Photocopying
Single photocopies of single articles may be made for personal use as allowed by national copyright laws. Permission of the Publisher and payment of a fee is required for all other photocopying, including multiple or systematic copying, copying for advertising or promotional purposes, resale, and all forms of document delivery. Special rates are available for educational institutions that wish to make photocopies for non-profit educational classroom use. For information on how to seek permission visit www.elsevier.com/permissions or call: (+44) 1865 843830 (UK)/(+1) 215 239 3804 (USA).

Derivative Works
Subscribers may reproduce tables of contents or prepare lists of articles including abstracts for internal circulation within their institutions. Permission of the Publisher is required for resale or distribution outside the institution. Permission of the Publisher is required for all other derivative works, including compilations and translations (please consult www.elsevier.com/permissions).

Electronic Storage or Usage
Permission of the Publisher is required to store or use electronically any material contained in this periodical, including any article or part of an article (please consult www.elsevier.com/permissions). Except as outlined above, no part of this publication may be reproduced, stored in a retrieval system or transmitted in any form or by any means, electronic, mechanical, photocopying, recording or otherwise, without prior written permission of the Publisher.

Notice
No responsibility is assumed by the Publisher for any injury and/or damage to persons or property as a matter of products liability, negligence or otherwise, or from any use or operation of any methods, products, instructions or ideas contained in the material herein. Because of rapid advances in the medical sciences, in particular, independent verification of diagnoses and drug dosages should be made.

Although all advertising material is expected to conform to ethical (medical) standards, inclusion in this publication does not constitute a guarantee or endorsement of the quality or value of such product or of the claims made of it by its manufacturer.

Otolaryngologic Clinics of North America (ISSN 0030-6665) is published bimonthly by Elsevier, Inc., 360 Park Avenue South, New York, NY 10010-1710. Months of issue are February, April, June, August, October, and December. Business and Editorial Offices: 1600 John F. Kennedy Blvd., Suite 1800, Philadelphia, PA 19103-2899. Customer Service Office: 6277 Sea Harbor Drive, Orlando, FL 32887-4800. Periodicals postage paid at New York, NY and additional mailing offices. Subscription prices are $450.00 per year (US individuals), $1336.00 per year (US institutions), $100.00 per year (US & Canadian student/resident), $576.00 per year (Canadian individuals), $1396.00 per year (Canadian institutions), $628.00 per year (international individuals), $1396.00 per year (international institutions), $270.00 per year (international student/resident). Foreign air speed delivery is included in all *Clinics'* subscription prices. All prices are subject to change without notice. **POSTMASTER:** Send address changes to *Otolaryngologic Clinics of North America*, Elsevier Health Sciences Division, Subscription Customer Service, 3251 Riverport Lane, Maryland Heights, MO 63043. **Telephone: 1-800-654-2452 (U.S. and Canada); 314-447-8871 (outside U.S. and Canada). Fax: 314-447-8029. E-mail: journalscustomerservice-usa@elsevier.com (for print support); journalsonlinesupport-usa@elsevier.com (for online support).**

Reprints. For copies of 100 or more of articles in this publication, please contact the Commercial Reprints Department, Elsevier Inc., 360 Park Avenue South, New York, NY 10010-1710. Tel.: 212-633-3874; Fax: 212-633-3820; E-mail: reprints@elsevier.com.

Otolaryngologic Clinics of North America is also published in Spanish by McGraw-Hill Interamericana Editores S.A., P.O. Box 5-237, 06500 Mexico D.F., Mexico.

Otolaryngologic Clinics of North America is covered in *MEDLINE/PubMed (Index Medicus), Current Contents/Clinical Medicine, Excerpta Medica, BIOSIS, Science Citation Index,* and *ISI/BIOMED.*

Contributors

CONSULTING EDITOR

SUJANA S. CHANDRASEKHAR, MD, FACS, FAAOHNS
Consulting Editor, Otolaryngologic Clinics of North America, Past President, American Academy of Otolaryngology-Head and Neck Surgery, Secretary-Treasurer, American Otological Society, Partner, ENT & Allergy Associates, LLP, Clinical Professor, Department of Otolaryngology-Head and Neck Surgery, Zucker School of Medicine at Hofstra-Northwell, Hempstead, Clinical Associate Professor, Department of Otolaryngology-Head and Neck Surgery, Icahn School of Medicine at Mount Sinai, New York, New York, USA

EDITORS

REGINA RODMAN, MD
Owner, Face Forward, Private Practice, Houston, Texas, USA

C. MICHAEL HABEN, MD, MSc
Director, Center for the Care of the Professional Voice, Haben Practice for Voice & Laryngeal Laser Surgery, PLLC, Rochester, New York, USA

AUTHORS

CHRISTELLA ANTONI, MSc, BA Hons, HCPC, MRCSLT, MASLTIP
Voice Specialist Speech and Language Therapist, Independent Practitioner, Visiting Lecturer in Transgender Voice, University College London (UCL), Chinese University of Hong Kong (CUHK), Voice Specialist SLT, Voice & Speech Services, Harrow, Middlesex, United Kingdom

JESÚS BÁEZ-MÁRQUEZ, MD
Board Certified by Mexican Council of Otolaryngology Head and Neck Surgery, Member of European Academy of Facial Plastic Surgery, Member of Mexican Society of Facial Plastic Surgery, Member of Spanish Society of Facial Plastic surgery, Member of Hospital Puerta de Hierro Andares, Zapopan, Jalisco, Mexico

SABRINA BRODY-CAMP, MD, MPH
Department of Otolaryngology–Head and Neck Surgery, Boston University School of Medicine, Boston, Massachusetts, USA; The Spiegel Center, Newton, Massachusetts, USA

PETER M. DEBBANEH, MD
Department of Head and Neck Surgery, Kaiser Permanente Medical Center at Oakland, Oakland, California, USA

ARUSHI GULATI, BS
Division of Facial Plastic and Reconstructive Surgery, Department of Otolaryngology–
Head and Neck Surgery, University of California, San Francisco, San Francisco,
California, USA

C. MICHAEL HABEN, MD, MSc
Director, Center for the Care of the Professional Voice, Haben Practice for Voice &
Laryngeal Laser Surgery, PLLC, Rochester, New York, USA

AMELIA ZHEANNA HUFF, BA
Educator at TransVoiceLessons and Internal Bioacoustics LLC, Clinton, Indiana, USA

JEFFREY S. JUMAILY, MD
Jeffrey Jumaily Facial Plastic Surgery, Los Angeles, California, USA

ANDREW J. KLEINBERGER, MD
Department of Head and Neck Surgery, Kaiser Permanente Walnut Creek Medical
Center, Walnut Creek, California, USA

P. DANIEL KNOTT, MD
Professor, Division of Facial Plastic and Reconstructive Surgery, Department of
Otolaryngology–Head and Neck Surgery, University of California, San Francisco, San
Francisco, California USA

HARRISON H. LEE, MD, DMD, FACS
Facial Plastic Surgery – Private Practice, Beverly Hills, California, USA; Facial Plastic
Surgery – Private Practice, New York, New York, USA

ANASTASIYA V. LYUBCHENKO, MD
Department of Oncology, Radiotherapy and Plastic Surgery, I.M. Sechenov First Moscow
State Medical University, Moscow, Russia

AINA M. MAGOMEDOVA, MD
Surgeon, FACEMAKER, Moscow, Russia

BRIAN A. NUYEN, MD
Voice Doctor Clinic, Stanford Otolaryngology–Head and Neck Surgery

BRYAN ROLFES, MD
Pinnacle Cosmetic, Wayzata, Minnesota, USA

NAHIR J. ROMERO, MD
Advanced Plastic Surgery, Washington, DC, USA

RAHUL SETH, MD
Associate Professor, Division of Facial Plastic and Reconstructive Surgery, Department of
Otolaryngology–Head and Neck Surgery, University of California, San Francisco, San
Francisco, California USA

JENNIFER N. SHEHAN, MD
Department of Otolaryngology–Head and Neck Surgery, Boston University School of
Medicine, Boston, Massachusetts, USA

MANSHER SINGH, MD
New York, New York, USA; Beverly Hills, California, USA

ANNA V. SLUZKY, MD
Surgeon, FACEMAKER, Moscow, Russia

MICHAEL SOMENEK, MD
Advanced Plastic Surgery, Washington, DC, USA

JEFFREY H. SPIEGEL, MD
Professor, Chief of Facial Plastic and Reconstructive Surgery, Department of
Otolaryngology–Head and Neck Surgery, Boston University School of Medicine, Boston,
Massachusetts, USA; The Spiegel Center, Newton, Massachusetts, USA

ANGELA STURM, MD, FACS
Private Practice, Assistant Clinical Professor, Department of Otolaryngology–Head and
Neck Surgery, University of Texas Medical Branch, Galveston, Texas, USA

CHRISTOPHER G. TANG, MD
Department of Head and Neck Surgery, Kaiser Permanente San Francisco Medical
Center, San Francisco, California, USA

CVETAN TASKOV, MD
Praxis für Plastische und Ästhetische Chirurgie Erding, Angermair-Haus, Erding, Germany

JAMES PHILLIP THOMAS, MD
Voice Doctor Clinic, Fellowship Director, Private Practice, Portland, Oregon, USA

Contents

**Approach to the Transgender Patient: Preoperative Counseling, Setting
Expectations, Avoiding Potential Postoperative Pitfalls**   707

Sabrina Brody-Camp, Jennifer N. Shehan, and Jeffrey H. Spiegel

An increasing number of transgender patients are seeking gender-affirming facial surgery, also known as facial feminization surgery. Physicians offering these services must be well versed in how to compassionately care for this patient population. We recommend having a well-informed staff that is knowledgeable about proper verbiage, use of pronouns, and preferred names for transgender patients. We also recommend helping patients to manage expectations and seek realistic goals from the first consultation. A frank discussion about the limits of facial feminization is essential. Discussing the prolonged recovery and expected outcome is of paramount importance preoperatively to avoid postoperative disappointment.

**Gender-Affirming Hormone Therapy: What the Head and Neck Surgeon Should
Know**   715

C. Michael Haben

The use of gender-affirming hormone therapy is found almost universally in transgendered and nonbinary patients presenting for gender-affirming surgical procedures of the face, neck, and voice. Surgeons caring for this population need to be aware of the effects, reasonable expectations, and limitations as well as potential perioperative risks of both continuation and discontinuation of hormone therapy.

**Modern Responses to Traditional Pitfalls in Gender Affirming Behavioral Voice
Modification**   727

Amelia Zheanna Huff

Gender-affirming behavioral voice modification has primarily been directed by cisgender clinicians who do not actively live or master the process of voice modification themselves but instead observe it from the outside looking in. The lack of a "lived experience" by cisgender instructors naturally leaves gaps and oversights that may reduce the effective potential of voice training. Input from transgender people who have learned voice modifications techniques is key to providing the best possible care. Ear training, direct vocal modeling, and mastery of gender-

affirmation throughout the United States. With growing trainee interest, program and fellowship director-related efforts to expand training, and progressive arcs of social change focusing on protections and promotion of TNG health, the future of OHNS training opportunities to serve TNG patients is promising.

The face is central to individual identity and gender presentation. Sex-based differences are seen at nearly every component of the face, from craniofacial structure to skin and soft tissue distribution. This article provides a framework for identification and analysis of sex-based differences in facial anatomy. This can then be used to guide individualized approaches to surgical planning to create greater congruence between patients' existing physical features and goals for gender expression.

 Video content accompanies this article at http://www.oto.theclinics.com.

Testosterone creates several characteristic changes in the upper face. These changes include elevating and squaring the hairline, flattening the central forehead, and increasing the anterior projection of the brow bone and orbital rims. When present, these changes will give a strong masculine characteristic to the face overall. Several techniques will be described here to restore the feminine characteristics of the upper face.

If the eyes are considered by some as the windows to the soul, the eyebrows can then be the frames that adorn them and can help accentuate a person's facial features. They are a staple of attractiveness, conveying emotion and projecting personality traits. Therefore, the utmost attention and intimate understanding of their role is required when modifying them to achieve an esthetically pleasing result. When discussing gender affirmation surgery, the eyebrows play a key role. In this article, we will discuss the important features and different approaches to achieve these modifications.

Facial gender affirmation surgery is currently growing worldwide and is an important treatment for gender dysphoria that will improve quality of life. The most frequently sought modifications by transgender women are forehead and supraorbital ridge reduction, cheek augmentation, upper lip surgery (lip lift), laryngeal chondroplasty, jaw reduction, and rhinoplasty. Rhinoplasty for transgender women uses the same techniques as rhinoplasty for a cisgender patient. However, knowledge of transgender care

a smooth transition from the ramus to the chin and also retains the integrity of the inner portion of the mandible. We discuss our techniques of jaw reduction surgery in this article.

Chondrolaryngoplasty is a well-described surgical procedure most commonly performed as part of facial feminization surgery for transgender patients with a diagnosis of gender dysphoria. A complete understanding of relevant neck anatomy and laryngeal function is critical to optimizing surgical outcomes. The overall goal of the procedure is to maximally reduce the thyroid cartilage prominence while preserving laryngeal integrity and minimizing the risk of external scarring. Among available approaches, the bronchoscopic-assisted technique with intraoperative needle localization has been demonstrated to reliably lead to safe and effective surgical outcomes while minimizing the risk of postoperative complications.

Conception of feminine face includes many different points, one of them is the hairline pattern, which is an important feature of gender identification. Here, we describe our utilization of 3D–modeling techniques in perioperative planning.

OTOLARYNGOLOGIC CLINICS
OF NORTH AMERICA

SERIES OF RELATED INTEREST

Facial Plastic Surgery Clinics
Available at: https://www.facialplastic.theclinics.com/

THE CLINICS ARE AVAILABLE ONLINE!
Access your subscription at:
www.theclinics.com

Foreword

Gender Affirmation in Otolaryngology: Compassion and Techniques

KEYWORDS

• Gender affirmation • Transgender • Otolaryngologic surgery

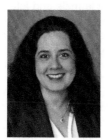

Sujana S. Chandrasekhar, MD, FACS, FAAOHNS
Consulting Editor

Shakespeare was wrong. A rose by another name does not smell as sweet, if the rose is a human who has been born into the wrong type of body. *Cisgender* (coined in the 1990s) refers to people whose gender identity matches what they were assigned at birth. *Transgender* (coined in the 1960s) refers to people who identify as a different gender than that which was assigned to them at birth. Trans people may experience dysphoria, a particular kind of existential anxiety that stems from not feeling like themselves, and they may or may not have surgery to affirm their gender. *Nonbinary* is a catch-all term for those whose gender identity does not fit within the traditional binary of man and woman.[1] None of these terms address the individual's sexuality, be it heterosexual, homosexual, or otherwise. About 1.6 million adults (over 18) and youth (aged 13 to 17) in the United States identify as transgender.[2] Three-quarters of them experience their first gender dysphoria by age 7. Transmen and transwomen live for a mean of 22.9 (SD 12.6) and 27.1 (SD 16.4) years, respectively, with untreated gender dysphoria before commencing nonsurgical gender transition.[3] Surgical interventions for gender affirmation can occur later.

The Trevor Project surveys 34,000 LGBTQ (lesbian, gay, bisexual, transgender, queer) youth aged 13 to 24 years annually, 48% of whom are transgender/nonbinary.[4] Of LGBTQ youth, 45% seriously considered attempting suicide in the past year; one in 5 transgender or nonbinary youth actually did attempt suicide. However, children and adolescents who are transgender are 50% less likely to attempt suicide if they have high social support from their family versus those who have low or no support. Fewer than one-third of transgender and nonbinary youth found their home to be gender-affirming. Support from family and caregivers includes the use of their preferred pronouns (he/she/they are the most commonly used ones) and their preferred name. In fact, the birth name is called their "dead" name, and it is hurtful to them to be called that name. People who are trans and/or nonbinary are not somehow choosing this path; this is who they are. They are not choosing ridicule and hate and ostracism; they are doing all that they can to live as who they actually are.

Although transgender issues have recently been subsumed into political discourse, most of it unkind and uncivil, the idea of gender fluidity is centuries old. In Hindu mythology, Lord Shiva is depicted as Ardhanarishvara, with half female and half male characteristics from head to toe, with the right side male and left side female. This extends to the style of eye, brow, cheek, lips, jaw, and neck as well as the rest of the body. Separately, Lord Vishnu comes to Earth as (not disguised as) Mohini, a beautiful woman whose weapon is Maya (illusion) to beguile and trick demons to save humanity and divinity.[5] Hermaphrodites of Greek mythology, the child of Hermes and Aphrodite, is depicted with both male and female features, usually female thighs, breasts, and style of hair, and male genitalia. The term "hermaphrodite," however, is considered a slur to intersex people. Another important character in Greek mythology is Tiresias, who is interestingly liminal, as he acts as a go-between for humans and the gods, has been both blind and seeing, and male and female, and can understand both the present and future at once.[6] Men have played women's parts in performances throughout civilizations, and women have had to live as men just to be able to follow their passions, be it doctoring (such as Dr James Barry, who was born Margaret Anne Bulkley), religious studies (Isaac Bashevis Singer's short story "Yentl the Yeshiva Boy"), writing (the famous French author Amantine Lucile Aurore Dupin, who wrote as George Sand and regularly wore men's clothing), and so forth.

When people think of gender-affirmation medicine and surgery, they often focus exclusively on hormonal therapy and genitourinary and mammary surgical intervention. However, our ability to project ourselves as who we are includes our face, neck, and voice. Subtle alterations, in the hands of skilled otolaryngologists and the talents of experienced speech and language pathologists and cosmetologists and other ancillary personnel, provide extraordinary quality-of-life improvements. Drs Rodman and Haben have put together a comprehensive issue of *Otolaryngologic Clinics of North America* on Gender-Affirmation Surgery in Otolaryngology. They begin with assessment and counseling and provide us with the tools to offer compassionate care to these patients who need it desperately. This type of surgical care cannot be delivered without full appreciation of the psychological and emotional aspects of the patient and their family's psyche and experience. Subsequent articles go through each aspect of Otolaryngologic care that can facilitate the change to masculine or feminine features and voice.

Every one of us entered medicine with the aim to help others, particularly in their time of need. Transgender men and women often face discrimination, bigotry, and hatred from their families, friends, and coworkers. These harsh reactions usually stem from fear and a basic misunderstanding of the transgender community. As physicians, it is our responsibility and our privilege to learn about, understand, and support these patients, their families, and our communities in seeing the humanity in each individual. I hope that as you read this issue of *Otolaryngologic Clinics of North America* in detail, you will feel the same way. If you would like to learn more about the LGBTQ community, please watch Episode 46 of my video show, She's On Call at https://youtu.be/Nth_ddFqR-U.

Sujana S. Chandrasekhar, MD, FACS, FAAOHNS
Consulting Editor
Otolaryngologic Clinics of North America

Past President
American Academy of Otolaryngology–
Head and Neck Surgery

Secretary-Treasurer and President-Elect
American Otological Society

Eastern Section Vice President and Sections Meeting Program Chair
Triological Society

Partner, ENT & Allergy Associates LLP
18 East 48th Street, 2nd Floor, New York, NY 10017, USA

Clinical Professor
Department of Otolaryngology– Head and Neck Surgery
Zucker School of Medicine at Hofstra–Northwell
Hempstead, NY, USA

Clinical Associate Professor
Department of Otolaryngology–Head and Neck Surgery
Icahn School of Medicine at Mount Sinai
New York, NY, USA

Co-Host and Co-Executive Producer
She's On Call

E-mail address:
ssc@nyotology.com

REFERENCES

1. Bateman, S. Cis, trans, nonbinary: A guide to gender terminology. Newshub, Dec 21, 2018. https://www.newshub.co.nz/home/lifestyle/2018/12/cis-trans-nonbinary-a-guide-to-gender-terminology.html. Accessed June 10, 2022.

2. Herman JL, Flores AR, O'Neill KK. (2022) How Many Adults and Youth Identify as Transgender in the United States? The Williams Institute, UCLA School of Law.

3. Zaliznyak M, Bresee C and Garcia MM. Age at first experience of gender dysphoria among transgender adults seeking gender-affirming surgery, JAMA Netw Open, 3 (3), 2020, e201236.

4. The Trevor Project National Survey on LGBTQ Youth Mental Health. https://www.thetrevorproject.org/survey-2022/assets/static/trevor01_2022survey_final.pdf. Accessed June 10, 2022.

5. Mohini: The Enchantress. American Institute of Indian Studies, Centre for Art and Archaeology. https://artsandculture.google.com/story/mohini-the-enchantress-

american-institute-of-indian-studies/pQXBuABQJikplg?hl=en. Accessed June 10, 2022.

6. Conway, M. Six Transgender Myths From Ancient Greece - And Are They Really Trans? https://paxsies.com/blogs/blogs-paxsies/greek-transgender-myths. Accessed June 10, 2022.

Preface

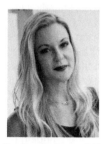 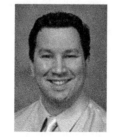

Regina Rodman, MD   C. Michael Haben, MD, MSc
Editors

In the United States, 1.4 million adults identify as transgender per a report published in 2016.[1,2] The actual number of transgender or nonbinary individuals is likely much higher, given that many do not self-report due to fear of stigmatization and discrimination. Considering the large number of gender-nonconforming individuals in the United States and across the world, it is highly likely that these patients will present to our offices for health care. Even those otolaryngologists who do not perform gender-affirming surgeries will certainly see these patients for complaints of the ear, nose, and throat unrelated to gender identity. Some of these patients may even be having general ENT issues due to treatments or procedures they have undertaken as part of their transition. It is necessary to treat these patients with dignity and respect. Some of these treatments, particularly hormone therapy, may have been obtained via the Internet and without the guidance of a medical professional. This is not uncommon in this population, where access to (compassionate) care may be lacking or absent. The goal of this issue is to provide a working knowledge of gender-affirming health care for otolaryngologists and allied health professionals.

We are living in an era of unprecedented political, social, and religious hyperpartisanship. Social media amplifies these divides and becomes an echo chamber instantaneously distributed to millions of subscribers on both sides of the divide. Laws are being enacted at the State level pitting physicians against the best interest of their patients and compliance with new anti-LGBTQ criminal statutes. When we became physicians and allied health professionals, we took an oath to "do no harm." This oath should supersede personal political, social, or religious views. Our primary commitment is to care for patients. In the care of gender-nonconforming patients, there are several ways we can fulfill this oath. The first is by creating a safe, LGBTQ-compassionate practice. This includes a basic understanding of sex versus gender identity, use of appropriate language, preferred pronouns and names, as well as an awareness of the biases, outright discrimination, and harassment this marginalized population has likely experienced in and out of the health care setting. The second is by becoming educated on gender-nonconforming specific health care, including hormone therapy, as well as gender-affirming surgeries of the head and neck, by understanding how

Otolaryngol Clin N Am 55 (2022) xvii–xviii
https://doi.org/10.1016/j.otc.2022.05.005
0030-6665/22/© 2022 Published by Elsevier Inc.   oto.theclinics.com

such treatment may be impacting the general ENT problems for which the patient might be seeking medical attention.

This population still faces daily discrimination and is often reluctant to seek health care due to previous damaging experiences. Suicide ideation is approximately 41% in transgender people compared with 4.6% in the average population. Suicidality may go up to more than 60% if the patient has a nonaffirming physician or the physician misgenders them. Treating these patients with trans-competent care is a matter of life and death. Sadly, the burden of education is often placed on the patient. This lack of confidence in the health care provider tends not only to scar patients but also may cause them to turn away from traditional medicine altogether in favor of more supportive, nontraditional alternative sources of treatments, including the dark Web.

We hope that in the articles to follow, the reader will gain a basic understanding of how to approach gender-nonconforming patients, gender-affirming hormone therapy, behavioral voice modification and speech therapy, laryngeal surgery for both trans-masculine and trans-feminine patients, tuning and refinements for voice, as well as descriptions of the procedures that are combined in facial feminization surgery.

www.professionalvoice.org (C.M. Haben)www.faceforwardhouston.com (R. Rodman)

Regina Rodman, MD
Face Forward
1900 North Loop West
Suite 370
Houston, TX 77018, USA

C. Michael Haben, MD, MSc
Center for the Care of the Professional Voice
Haben Practice for Voice &
Laryngeal Laser Surgery, PLLC
980 Westfall Road
Building 100, Suite 127
Rochester, NY 14618, USA

E-mail addresses:
dr.rodman@faceforwardhouston.com (R. Rodman)
Michael.Haben.MD@professionalvoice.org (C.M. Haben)

REFERENCES

1. Available at: http://williamsinstitute.law.ucla.edu/wp-content/uploads/How-Many-Adults-Identify-as-Transgender-in-the-United-States.pdf.
2. AMA Policy: reducing suicide risk among lesbian, gay, bisexual, transgender, and questioning youth through collaboration with allied organizations H-60.927.

Approach to the Transgender Patient

Preoperative Counseling, Setting Expectations, Avoiding Potential Postoperative Pitfalls

Sabrina Brody-Camp, MD, MPH[a,b], Jennifer N. Shehan, MD[a], Jeffrey H. Spiegel, MD[a,b],*

KEYWORDS

- Transgender • Facial surgery • Facial feminization surgery • Preoperative counseling

KEY POINTS

- There is the rising incidence of patients seeking gender-affirming facial surgery (facial feminization surgery).
- Providers performing facial feminization need an understanding of psychosocial considerations related to transgender medical care.
- All staff caring for transgender patients should be well versed in the care of this population including using appropriate verbiage, pronouns, and preferred names.
- The surgeon must determine specifically what each patient's goals are in terms of degree of femininity desired as well as specific areas of concern.
- It is essential that patients are aware of the limitations of facial feminization surgery. There is no guarantee that surgery will change how they perceive themselves or how others perceive them.

INTRODUCTION

There may be more than 1.4 million people in the United States who identify as transgender based on the limited epidemiologic studies performed for this population.[1-3] An increasing number of people openly identify as transgender, and government at both the state and federal level has rightfully proposed more legal protection for this group.[4] With higher visibility in the health care setting, there is more emphasis on standards for treatment of transgender patients.[5]

[a] Department of Otolaryngology – Head and Neck Surgery, Boston University School of Medicine, One Boston Medical Center Place, Boston, MA 02118, USA; [b] The Spiegel Center, 335 Boylston Street, Newton, MA 02459, USA
* Corresponding author. The Spiegel Center, 335 Boylston Street, Newton, MA 02459, USA
E-mail address: info@DrSpiegel.com

Otolaryngol Clin N Am 55 (2022) 707–713
https://doi.org/10.1016/j.otc.2022.04.001
0030-6665/22/© 2022 Elsevier Inc. All rights reserved.
oto.theclinics.com

Appropriate terminology use regarding transgender patients is critical. "Sex" (male or female) refers to the internal and external sex organs, chromosomes, and hormonal activities within the body as assigned at birth. "Gender" is accepted to be defined socially, culturally, and personally by the individual. The preferred definitions within this category continue to evolve. Although a spectrum of gender is described by experts, including "nonbinary" individuals, it is primarily transgender women who seek facial plastic surgery. Transgender male, or female-to-male transition, refers to a person who was assigned female at birth but identifies as a man or on the masculine spectrum.[6] Transgender female, or male-to-female transition, refers to a person who was assigned male at birth but identifies as a woman or on the feminine spectrum. Gender-affirming surgery has become a popular title used to describe the surgical procedures that are potentially beneficial for transgender patients. Transgender men seeking facial masculinization are quite rare; over the last 22 years, the senior author has only seen a handful of transgender patients seeking masculinization. For this reason, this article will largely be focused on patients seeking facial feminization surgery (FFS).

A distinction should also be made between gender nonconformity and gender dysphoria. Gender nonconformity refers to the difference between an individual's gender identity, role, or expression compared with the cultural normative assigned to their sex.[7] Based on the Diagnostic and Statistical Manual of Mental Disorders— 5th edition, gender dysphoria is a discrepancy between a person's gender identity and a person's sex, which leads to a significant change in social, occupational, or other areas of functioning.[8,9] Patients with gender dysphoria feel limited in their ability to function in society because of the incongruity of their gender identity and their physical appearance. These are the individuals who often seek out gender-affirming surgeries. Gender nonconformity does not necessitate gender dysphoria; individuals who are gender nonconforming and are satisfied with their appearance are generally not those that present to our office.

Transgender patients are less likely to have health insurance coverage compared with the general population.[10,11] With a lack of insurance also comes lack of coverage for treatments such as hormone therapy and gender-affirming surgery.[12] Nonetheless, the number of patients presenting for gender-related surgical care continues to increase.[13] This may be related to the Affordable Care Act, which prevented insurance carriers from excluding health services related to "gender transition."

Surgical procedures in the head and neck aimed to create more feminine features, known collectively as FFS, are challenging in terms of the wide array of techniques and skills necessary for a successful outcome but rewarding in the ability to significantly improve quality of life.[14] Physicians who facilitate gender transition have the opportunity to enhance the lives of transgender patients by making an impact on both physical appearance and psychosocial well-being.[7] We describe a set of important considerations when seeing transgender patients in consultation for facial feminization. We hope that our experience will help to avoid postoperative pitfalls and arrive at an outcome that is favorable to both the patient and surgeon.

DISCUSSION

Excellent care of a transgender patient begins before the patient even enters the office. Clinical staff must be trained in how to greet transgender persons, and the importance of appropriate language should be stressed. Continuous reinforcement and education of the office, operating room, and hospital staff can lead to a more inclusive and comfortable environment. Problematic terms like "biologically male" "genetically female," and "cross-dresser" should be avoided. Naturally, defamatory language including "deceptive," "masquerading," "posing," "tranny," "she male," and "he/she" are not to be tolerated.[15]

Addressing a transgender patient by their chosen name and preferred pronoun is often the first step in establishing a trusting doctor–patient relationship. Those who are frequently misgendered appreciate an environment where they feel accepted. A patient's preferred pronouns and name should be determined from first contact and documented in the patient's chart before their arrival for consultation. When a patient calls to schedule a consultation for gender affirmation surgery, the receptionist booking the appointment will pointedly ask their preferred pronouns and name. If a mistake is made at any point in consultation, apologize with sincerity, and from then on make a point of addressing them correctly.

Even with adequate staff familiarity of appropriate vocabulary, a patient's name and pronouns can be challenging in the health care setting. Although some patients are comfortable being referred to by their birth name, most of the transgender patients prefer their chosen name. This can become particularly challenging with regards to consents and prescriptions. It is our practice to ask patients to provide both their legal name (what is written on their legal identification) and preferred name. If these names differ, we ask that they write both on their consent forms—both their legal name and the "correct" name. Although some transgender patients have legally changed their identification to match their preferred name and pronouns, others have not. It is important to have an open conversation about these matters before prescribing medication or consenting a patient, as to avoid confusion or dissatisfaction when a patient is picking up a prescription or having a procedure performed.

When treating this unique patient population, it is important to remember your intentions to help patients and ease suffering. In addition, it is assumed that each physician wants to practice in an atmosphere of excellence with unparalleled experience and outcomes for their patients. Using patient-preferred names and pronouns is a very simple but important part of creating that environment. Again, it can be helpful to ask patients to use their "driver's license" name on legal documents but to write their preferred name next to that (or above). People understand the use of legal names on legal documents without taking offense. You can also tell them to use their legal name even if it is an old name that they have not gotten around to changing yet. This statement reveals that you respect both their identity and the important legal aspects of our profession.

Preoperative Counseling

Most of the transgender patients who seek consultation at our office are trans female and are seeking feminizing procedures. The remainder of the discussion relates specifically to these patients and procedures that are under the umbrella of gender-affirming facial surgery/ FFS.

When a patient arrives to our office in consultation for FFS, our approach is always the same. We start by speaking about where they live, what they do, or other interesting aspects of their life. This relaxes the frequently anxious patient and demonstrates that we see them as a person, not as a transgender patient. After establishing a relaxed rapport, we ask the patient to first look in a mirror and discuss what areas they specifically would like to address. At the same time, we write down a list of procedures that we feel would benefit them in looking more feminine. Afterward, we see how the surgeon and patient "matchup" by comparing the patient's desired changes and the list of procedures suggested by the surgeon. This process allows the patient to feel autonomous, and they have gotten the chance to bring up any area of concern. The exercise also permits the surgeon to point out specific procedures that perhaps the patient was not aware could be affecting their femininity and perceived gender. Each aspect of the proposed surgical plan is described including incision locations, recovery times, and potential complications. When options exist, the patient is presented with the choices and our recommendation, but given the opportunity to choose what she prefers.

As with any elective surgery, it is imperative to recognize patients that have unrealistic expectations early on. This requires a delicate balance and ultimately is on the onus of the surgeon to explain what is possible and what is not. We encourage patients to bring in pictures of others or ideal outcomes that can help guide us in our surgical planning. Pictures of close relatives (eg, mother, sister) are particularly helpful as they are more likely to be achievable than photos of models or celebrities. Also, family photos help the surgeon to understand the type of outcome that the patient will find satisfactory. On the other hand, we have had patients provide anime characters or other highly edited photos as a desired final outcome. Politely and respectfully, we must explain why this is simply not possible with any amount of surgery. In addition, it is not uncommon for 65 year old transgender women to show heavily stylized photos of 19 year old models as the preferred outcome. In these situations, we bluntly explain that the result is not possible and that our idea of a successful outcome would be for them to look like a 60-year-old woman or, put another way, the grandmother of the person in the photo.

Not every patient seeking facial feminization is necessarily trying to look as feminine as possible all of the time. Some patients are at a point in their transition where they would like to pick and choose which settings they feel comfortable appearing more feminine, while in others retaining a male identity. For instance, they may still be presenting as male at work or to their family, whereas the remainder of the time they present as female. Of course, many others approach surgery with a mindset of hoping to appear the most feminine version of themselves at all times. Determining what the patient desires from surgery is essential to reaching an outcome that both the patient and surgeon are satisfied with.

Setting Expectations

Masculinity and femininity sit on a broad, multidimensional spectrum. How we define each end of the spectrum, "traditional" masculine and feminine concepts, relates to appearance as well as behavior. In our culture, we associate certain physical features, manners, interests, personality traits, and occupations with being inherently male or female.[16] As surgeons performing FFS, we can only change where a person sits on this spectrum to a certain degree. It is not possible to bring a person from one extreme end of the spectrum all the way to the other. In addition, as discussed previously, patients may not desire to move as far toward traditionally feminine as possible.

Our perception of an attractive feminine facial appearance is determined by several factors. First, feminine bony anatomy or "bone structure," includes a vertical, flat forehead with elevated eyebrows, high, prominent cheek bones, a narrow, small nose, a tapered jaw and chin, and a slender, smooth neck. A trait that is akin to femininity is youthfulness—diffuse rhytids, jowling, dermatochalasia, and a long cutaneous upper lip contribute to both looking older and more masculine. Hairless and flawless skin also intrinsically creates a more feminine appearance overall. A full head of hair is both youthful and associated with femininity. In addition to these features, a petite frame, breast tissue, and an hourglass figure also fit into the overall appearance of womanhood.

Although the physical appearance contributes significantly to how a person is gendered by society, several other factors come into play. How a person speaks can be associated with a specific gender. This included the pitch, volume, and tone of their voice but also their choice of words and manner of speaking. Similarly, the way in which a person carries themselves—walking, sitting, and hand gesturing—often has an effect on where they are perceived on the gender spectrum. How one chooses to dress is one of the simplest but most obvious indications of gender. Last, one's physical build—shoulder width, hips, and height—are inherent traits that are linked to a person's sex. All of these elements play a significant role in a patient's gender as perceived by others.

We make clear to patients that although we can successfully address several (though not all) aspects of their physical facial appearance to make them appear more feminine, we cannot necessarily change the more nuanced behavioral factors that also play into gender. In fact, every patient that undergoes facial feminization with our team must sign a consent explicitly stating this fact that surgery has no guarantee to change the way the patient or others perceive them. Some patients choose to opt for certain procedures and not others that we have suggested. We discuss with these patients that this may limit how far along the spectrum they can move toward more femininity.

Avoiding Postoperative Pitfalls

It is essential to discuss recovery and expectations for healing time at the first consultation. As we tell our patients, mandible contouring in particular has a slower recovery and delays the gratification of FFS. Similarly, hair grafts will not look their best for several months. If the patient has any major life events approaching or a job that requires looking a certain way on a daily basis, timing of surgery becomes exceedingly important.

We often give the analogy to patients of having surgery as like a pregnant person giving birth. After having a baby, the mother's abdomen does not immediately shrink back to its prepregnancy size. Similarly, after FFS, the complete effects of surgery take a period of weeks to months to be fully realized.

Most of our patients undergoing FFS return to the clinic the following day. This visit serves as both a practical postoperative check for complications and also an opportunity to provide reassurance. Patients are often quite edematous and bruised. If they have had mandible contouring their face is enlarged significantly more than preoperatively. We provide assurance that the first day after surgery is the worst in terms of pain and swelling, but that every day should get better. We typically see the patients again 1 week following surgery. At this point, we remove sutures and staples as needed and reiterate the expected recovery course. As many of our patients travel from afar, we do not have scheduled in person follow-up after the first week. We encourage patients to send photographs or set up virtual visits to keep us informed of their progress. Should any complication arise, we make sure to let patients know it would be best to see us in person to address them. Any concerns or questions are welcomed, and any patient who requests a visit is scheduled promptly. Patients need to know that they are safeguarded, and we communicate that after surgery we remain available to assist them as best we can for as long as they need us.

SUMMARY

FFS is becoming more popular as increasing numbers of transgender patients are seeking gender affirmation surgery. This unique patient group requires special considerations for preoperative counseling in order to optimize postoperative results. One must manage expectations ahead of surgery, especially when it comes to how others may perceive the patient's gender postoperatively. Ultimately, as with all patients, transgender patients deserve to be treated with dignity and respect. By taking the time to attend to their specific needs and goals, it is possible to achieve a successful outcome that provides immeasurable satisfaction for a transgender patient.

As a final thought, it is helpful to instill in both yourself as physician and your staff to recognize transgender patients as courageous. If given the choice, no one would choose to have gender dysphoria. It is a difficult and constant stress. Making the choice to rise and face the challenge, seek medical help, and undergo the many surgical and lifestyle changes necessary to transition is not easy. Many would, and have, chosen to suppress these feelings and live an unhappy life. We respect the strength necessary to conspicuously seek help, appreciate the opportunity to use our training to provide comfort to others, and hope that we would have similar courage if presented with such a challenge.

CLINICS CARE POINTS

- Increasing numbers of transgender patients are seeking gender affirmation surgery in the form of facial feminization.
- Approaching the transgender patient requires knowledge of appropriate verbiage, pronouns, and preferred names on the part of both the physician and staff.
- Establish early on what the specific goals are for each specific patient seeking facial feminization surgery (FFS).
- Manage expectations appropriately as FFS can only accomplish so much in adjusting a patient's perceived gender.
- Give adequate counseling in regards to prolonged recovery time and delayed gratification.
- Treating transgender patients with dignity and respect is crucial to achieving a satisfactory result.

DISCLOSURE

The authors have no commercial or financial conflicts of interest to disclose.

REFERENCES

1. Flores A, Herman J, Gates G, Brown T. How many adults identify as transgender in the United States? Los Angeles, CA: The Williams Institute; 2016.
2. Reisner S, Poteat T, Keatley J. Global health burden and needs of transgender populations: a review. Lancet 2016;388(10042):412–36.
3. Zucker K. Epidemiology of gender dysphoria and transgender identity. Sex Health 2017;14(5):404–11.
4. Minkin R, Brown A. Rising shares of U.S. adults know someone who is trasngender or goes by gender neutral pronouns. Washington, D.C.: Pew Research Center; 2021.
5. Clark J, Boyon N, Jackson C. Global attitudes toward transgender people. Paris, France: Ipsos; 2018.
6. Kuper L, Nussbaum R, Mustanski B. Exploring the diversity of gender and sexual orientation identities in an online sample of transgender individuals. J Sex Res 2012;49(2–3):244–54.

7. Spiegel JH. Challenges in Care of the Transgender Patient Seeking Facial Feminization Surgery. Facial Plast Surg Clin North Am 2008;16(2):233–8.
8. Coleman, E., Bockting W., Botzer M., et al. Standards of care for the health of transsexual, transgender, and gender nonconforming people. *International Journal of Transgenderism*. 13 (4), 2012, 165-232.
9. Davy Z, Toze M. What is gender dysphoria? A critical systematic narrative reivew. Transgend Health 2018;3(1):159–69.
10. Roberts T, Fantz C. Barriers to quality health care for the transgender population. Clin Biochem 2014;47(10–11):983–7.
11. Daniel H, Butkus R. Health and public policy committee of american college of physicians: lesbian, gay, bisexual, and transgender health disparities: executive summary of a policy position paper from the American college of physicians. Ann Intern Med 2015;163(2):135–7.
12. Lane M, Ives G, Sluiter E. Trends in gender-affirming surgery in insured patients in the United States. Plast Reconstr Surg Glob Open 2018;6(4):e1738.
13. Murad M, Elamin M, Garcia M. Hormonal therapy and sex reassignment: a systematic review and meta-analysis of quality of life and psychosocial outcomes. Clin Endocrinol 2010;62:214–31.
14. Spiegel JH. Facial Feminization for the Transgender Patient. J Craniofac Surg 2019;30(5):1399–402.
15. GLAAD Media Reference Guide – Transgender. Glossary of Terms – Transgender. Available at: http://www.glaad.org/reference/transgender. Accessed November 1, 2021.
16. Kachel S, Steffens M, Niedlich C. Traditional masculinity and femininity: validation of a a new scale assessing gender roles. Front Psychol 2016;7:956.

Gender-Affirming Hormone Therapy

What the Head and Neck Surgeon Should Know

C. Michael Haben, MD, MSc*

KEYWORDS

- Transgender • Nonbinary • Hormone • Feminization • Masculinization • Estrogen
- Testosterone

KEY POINTS

- Gender-affirming hormone therapy is present nearly universally in the transgender population.
- Understanding of the effects, expectations, limitations, and risks of hormone therapy is vital to optimal care of this population.
- Perioperative management of hormone therapy is an important aspect of surgical planning.

INTRODUCTION

Up to 3% of the US population identifies as transgendered/gender incongruent, nonbinary, or "other."[1] Transgender is defined as having a binary gender identity or expression that is the opposite from the one assigned at birth. In contrast, cis-gender is defined as having the same binary gender or expression that is assigned at birth.

There is a growing number of individuals who do not ascribe to a binary gender classification and consider themselves as nonbinary, a gender, gender neutral, gender bender, third gender, or androgynous. In 2016, New York City identified 31 different, officially recognized gender classifications.[2] Although feminizing or masculinizing gender-affirming hormone therapy (F-GAHT and M-GAHT) has historically been considered for those individuals who are transgender in a binary sense, it is increasingly being used for nonbinary individuals whose identity or expression is more feminine or masculine than the sex assigned at birth without being specifically "male" or "female."

The demographics of this population seem to be changing. In additional to a significant increase in the overall number of individuals self-reporting to this group, the

Center for the Care of the Professional Voice, 980 Westfall road, Suite 1-127, Rochester, NY 14618, USA
* Corresponding Author.
E-mail address: Michael.Haben.MD@professionalvoice.org

Otolaryngol Clin N Am 55 (2022) 715–726
https://doi.org/10.1016/j.otc.2022.04.002
0030-6665/22/© 2022 Elsevier Inc. All rights reserved.

oto.theclinics.com

mean age seeking initiation of hormone therapy has decreased steadily with the average age in both male and female dropping to less than 30 years at one institution[3] and a steady increase in the percentage of female-to-male (FTM) such that it is now equivalent to male-to-female (MTF). Regardless of specific prevalence rates, most studies demonstrate two clear trends: (1) growth in the proportion of gender noncon-forming self-identifying individuals over time and (2) a higher proportion of noncon-forming identities among the younger generations.[4] These findings may be due in part to increasing visibility, acceptance, and understanding of gender nonconforming individuals. Another important factor could be the move away from classifying gender incongruence as a mental disorder. In the latest Diagnostic and Scientific Manual and International Classification of Diseases "gender identity disorder" has been replaced with gender dysphoria (GD) and gender incongruence. GD is defined as a marked incongruence between one's experienced and/or expressed gender and assigned gender at birth.[5]

The American Psychiatry Association in a policy statement makes it important to note that gender nonconformity is not in itself a mental disorder.[6] This population, however, possesses a high prevalence of coexisting anxiety, depression, substance abuse, suicide, lower rates of health utilization, higher rates of tobacco use, obesity, sexually transmitted diseases , and HIV-infections compared with their cisgendered counterparts.[7,8]

There is some evidence that GD manifests commonly in early childhood, with a me-dian age of 6 years for both female and male transgendered individuals and could persist untreated for decades before individuals commence gender transition ther-apy.[9] There seems to be a movement to identify and treat GD in adolescents and youth earlier in pubertal development.[10] In this population subset, current hormonal regi-mens aim to achieve full pubertal suppression with the modulation of endogenous sex hormone effects in addition to the development of secondary sex characteristics congruent with the affirmed gender.[11] This trend may ultimately have a significant impact on the timing, feasibility, and practical and ethical considerations of gender-affirming surgery (GAS) of the head and neck for future generations for gender non-conforming youths.[12]

This article will look at some of the most common hormonal therapies used for gender transitioning and the state of research on how or how long a particular therapy might impact the timing of various components of gender confirming surgery in the head and neck.

GENDER-AFFIRMING HORMONAL THERAPY

For most transgendered individuals, accessing GAHT is a necessary and generally first step in their transition. The basic concept of GAHT is to replicate as closely as possible the hormone environment that is concordant with the person's gender iden-tity.[13] The primary endpoints of GAHT are to address the GD[14] (and secondarily improve the coexisting anxiety, substance abuse, suicidal ideation and depression, when present) and promote the secondary sex characteristics of the affirmed gender.

GAHT in accordance with current clinic practice guidelines is generally safe and effective.[15] Hormone therapy was traditionally used in patients with binary gender incongruence, that is, men transitioning to women or vice-versa. Recently, its use has broadened beyond transgendered individuals to include gender neutral, bigender, androgynous, nongender, and other individuals experiencing GD wishing to have sec-ondary sex characteristics more feminine or masculine than those they possess. Although some people may wish to achieve the greatest possible masculinization or feminization from hormonal interventions, others may only seek sufficient hormones to achieve an androgynous appearance.

Chemically synthesized estrogens and testosterone became commercially available in the 1930s and 1940s. It was not until 1979 that the first standards of care regarding hormonal therapy for transgendered individuals were developed. These standards eventually became an international organization of multidisciplinary trans-health professionals named The World Professional Association of Transgender Health (WPATH)[16] intending to be a global education initiative providing surgeons and other health care professionals the necessary background knowledge to understand and care for this unique population. The most recent updated Standards of Care version 8 is expected by the end of December 2021 at the time of this writing.[17] Additional clinical guidelines have been published by the Endocrinology Society[18] in the United States among others in Europe[19] and elsewhere.[20] Gender-transitioning patients would ideally be served by a multidisciplinary approach which includes providers in primary care, behavioral health, members of various surgical specialties and subspecialties, in addition to endocrinology. In most settings this idealized multidisciplinary approach is simply not practical or even available because of a myriad of barriers to access. More and more, primary care physicians are assuming the lead in the diagnosis of GD, initiation and routine testing of individuals on GAHT as well as screening and management of comorbidities.[21] An often overlooked aspect of care is how the timing of one therapy may impact the timing of subsequent therapies including gender affirmation surgery.

Coordination may be especially problematic when patients are treated by providers that are literally hundreds or thousands of miles away from other members of the team, in an unaffiliated center, or even located in a different country. The proportion of individuals in this population having to travel very long distances to access care, especially surgical specialists, is tremendous.[22]

GAHT may be broadly classified as either feminizing (F-GAHT) or masculinizing (M-GAHT). F-GAHT is based on the use of exogenous estrogen, alone or in various combinations[23] with the goal of increasing serum estradiol concentrations and decreasing serum testosterone concentrations into a range similar to cisgender premenopausal female *[Hembree 18]*,[24] When used in combination with estrogen, additional agents fall into four general categories: (1) progestins,[25] (2) androgen blockers including cyproterone and the antiandrogen spironolactone, (3) gonadotropin-releasing hormone agonists such as leuprolide, and (4) 5-alpha reductase inhibitors, typically finasteride.[26] If orchiectomy is completed (alone or as part of full gender affirmation "bottom" surgery), androgen-blockers and GnRH agonists are terminated.

Although a wide variety of hormone regimens have been developed, there are no published reports of randomized clinical trials comparing efficacy in producing physical transition.

Beyond ameliorating GD, the expectations for F-GAHT on secondary sex characteristics in adults are myriad and include enhancement of breast development, skin softening, slowing of androgenic hair loss, fat redistribution (from abdomen to hips), and reduction in testicular and prostate size. Feminizing GAHT has also been shown to decrease strength, lean body mass, and muscle area, effects considered to be desirable.[27] The most commonly cited secondary sex characteristic end point for F-GAHT is breast development.[28] In one study for transgender women, breast development was the most anticipated change in over 35% of respondents, followed by gynoid fat deposition.[29]

Testosterone is the mainstay of M-GAHT and can be administered via a nasal route, weekly subcutaneous/intramuscular injection or transdermal gel/patch. An oral route recently approved by the FDA for cisgendered men with medically low testosterone[30] may soon be available to transgendered men. The effects of M-GAHT on secondary sex characteristics include cessation of menses, facial hair development, deepening of the voice, clitoromegaly, fat redistribution from the hips to abdomen, oily skin, acne, and increased muscle mass and strength. The most commonly cited secondary sex characteristic end point for M-GAHT is cessation of menses.[31] Amenorrhea and a deeper voice were the secondary sex characteristic most anticipated in adults starting M-GAHT at 52.7% and 32.4%, respectively. Masculinizing GAHT improves GD, quality of life , and social functioning within 6 months of therapy. In contrast, transgendered females do not seem to gain the same early benefit from GAHT and seem to be more likely to require surgical procedures of the head and neck because of the relatively modest impacts of feminizing hormone regimens on highly noticeable secondary sex characteristics of the face and voice.[14]

Most physical changes, whether feminizing or masculinizing, occur over the course of 2 years. The amount of physical change and the exact timeline of effects can be highly variable. This can and should be taken into consideration when contemplating the age, timing, and candidacy of irreversible surgical procedures. A commonly cited approximate time course for physical changes[18] from initiation of F-GAHT are

- Breast growth expected by 3 to 6 months. Maximum benefit usually realized in 2 to 3 years.
- Gynoid body fat redistribution expected by 3 to 6 months. Maximum benefit usually realized in 2 to 5 years.
- Decreased lean body mass, strength, and muscle area expected by 3 to 6 months. Maximum benefit usually realized in 1 to 2 years.
- Skin softening expected by 3 to 6 months. Maximum benefit usually realized in 2 to 3 years.
- Slowed growth of body and facial hair expected by 3 to 6 months. Unknown time to maximum benefit because of the number of dermatologic procedures frequently undertaken.
- Slowed androgenic hair loss (male pattern baldness) expected at 1 to 3 months. Maximum benefit usually realized in 1 to 2 years; however, no regrowth of prior hair loss is expected.
- Voice: no changes are expected or observed.

And from initiation of M-GAHT are:

- Amenorrhea expected by 2 to 6 months. Maximum benefit usually realized in 1 to 2 years.
- Voice deepening expected by 3 to 12 months. Maximum benefit usually realized in 1 to 2 years.
- Facial and body hair virilization expected by 3 to 6 months. Maximized benefit usually realized in 3 to 5 years.
- Oily skin and acne expected at 1 to 6 months. Maximum benefit usually realized in 1 to 2 years.
- Androgenic hair loss expected at 1 to 6 months. Maximum benefit highly dependent on age and genetics.
- Increased muscle mass and strength expected at 6 to 12 months. Maximum benefit usually realized at 2 to 5 years
- Masculine body fat redistribution expected at 3 to 6 months. Maximum benefit usually realized in 2 to 5 years.

The degree to which these changes occur can vary greatly from person to person and may be dependent on the age at which GAHT is initiated, exact regimen prescribed, as well as the presence and impact of medical comorbidities. It should be noted that the hormone therapy, whether with estrogen or testosterone, is usually continued lifelong, even after oophorectomy or orchiectomy. Overall, adult transgendered men have a higher rate of achieving the head and neck secondary sex characteristics of their affirmed gender using M-GAHT than women using F-GAHT as testosterone therapy typically generates highly visible changes in the face (growth of facial hair, thickening of the skin, increase in frontal bossing, and so forth)[31] and voice.[32] Universally, F-GAHT makes less of a definitive difference in the face[33] with no real effect on facial beard and bony structure or the voice. Without realizing many of the secondary sex characteristics of cisgendered females on hormone therapy alone, transgender females frequently seek out facial feminization surgery, feminization laryngoplasty, and procedures for facial hair removal to address this disparity in GAHT.

Hembree[18] describes three categories or stages of physical interventions for GD:

Fully reversible interventions. These involve the use of GnRH analogues to suppress estrogen or testosterone production before gonad surgery and consequently limit the physical changes and development of secondary sex characteristics of their nonaffirmed gender due to puberty. This category is generally limited to adolescents and young adults who have not completed puberty or had gonad surgery.

Partially reversible interventions. These include GAHT to masculinize or feminize the body. Some hormone-induced changes may need reconstructive surgery to reverse the effect (eg, gynecomastia caused by estrogens or deepening of the voice caused by testosterone) should de-transition back to birth gender become necessary.

Irreversible interventions. These are surgical procedures, including most GAS procedures of the head and neck.

In adolescents, Hembree contends, a stepwise process is recommended to keep options open through the first two stages. Moving from one stage to another should not occur until there has been adequate time for adolescents and their parents to assimilate fully the effects of earlier interventions.

SURGICAL CANDIDACY

WPATH, in its most recent Standards of Care publication (SOC 7, published in 2012),[16] strongly recommended that patients considering genital ("bottom") surgery have not only a persistent, well-documented history of GD but also completed 12 continuous months of hormonal therapy. The SOC 7 rationale for a preoperative, 12-month experience of living in an identity-congruent gender role is based on expert clinical consensus that a year provides sufficient opportunity for most patients to experience and adjust to their affirmed gender role before considering a surgical procedure. Twelve months allow for a range of different life experiences and events that typically take place including family events, holidays, vacations, and etcetera. During this time, patients are encouraged to present themselves in their affirmed gender role consistently on a daily basis and across all settings of life. It has been recommended that this process includes disclosure to partners, family, friends, coworkers, and members of the individual's community.

Although there are no explicit recommendations in the SOC 7 for behavioral health documentation or duration of hormonal therapy before head and neck surgical procedures, some providers extrapolate WPATHs genital surgery recommendations including: living as the affirmed gender and on appropriate GAHT for a minimum of 1 year before considering an individual a reasonable candidate for irreversible surgery. Other providers report a small but not insignificant percentage of patients, notably male-to-female transgendered individuals, who present either not having initiated GAHT or electing not to pursue hormonal therapy because of a variety of reasons including maintenance of reproductive capabilities or reticence to endure the adverse effects of treatment. A 1-year waiting period and/or GAHT requirement could exacerbate already severe dysphoria, particularly male-to-female transgendered individuals where F-GAHT is not expected to significantly improve most of the visible secondary sex characteristics, namely the face and voice. As such, clinical judgment and an individualized approach would be prudent when extrapolating guidelines across surgical specialities and assessing surgical candidacy.

Although laryngeal and facial plastic procedures do not require referral by mental health providers, such professionals can play an important role assisting patients in making a fully informed decision about the timing and implications of such procedures in the context of the overall transition. Evaluation for psychological suitability for surgery could decrease the risk of postoperative depression or suicide as recovery from major surgery can be very stressful. Questions to be considered are (1) whether the patient has been on GAHT for a sufficient amount of time and with adequate support services to control the GD as much as medically possible allowing for true informed consent for an irreversible surgical procedure; (2) whether the duration of GAHT has been sufficient to permit the expected impact(s) to be fully realized; and (3) has the patient fully embraced their affirmed gender, including disclosure to their immediate circle, sufficient to provide adequate support during the postoperative recovery? This final consideration may be principally vital for patients who traveled hundreds (or thousands) of miles for a procedure and may return home postoperatively to less than ideal support systems.

PERIOPERATIVE GENDER-AFFIRMING HORMONE THERAPY

Gender-affirming surgical procedures of the head and neck invariably occur after starting hormone therapy. Hormone management in the perioperative period requires an understanding of the risks and benefits of GAHT as well as an understanding of risk-mitigation strategies. There are various deleterious effects associated with GAHT that could potentially play a role in perioperative surgical complications[34] including hypertrigliceridemia, hyperprolactinemia, and coronary artery disease on feminizing hormones; erythrocytosis, destabilization of certain psychiatric disorders and hypertension on masculinizing hormones; and weight gain, elevated liver enzymes and blood pressure changes associated with either hormone therapy. The most commonly cited concern with the use of F-GAHT both during and outside of the perioperative period is that of the risk of venous thromboembolism (VTE) due to estrogen. VTE is a known risk for certain formulations of estradiol therapy and is the most common side effect of F-GAHT reported.[18] It is important for surgeons to understand the perioperative risk of VTE and strategies to mitigate the chances of deep venous thrombosis, pulmonary embolism, myocardial infarction, and stroke. The VTE risks associated with exogenous hormones have well-studied in cisgender females on hormone replacement therapy, however, transgender females are unique in that they are typically on much higher doses of hormone therapy; start therapy much younger; and remain on it lifelong in most cases.[35] Extrapolating existing data on cisgender females taking hormonal replacement therapy may not appropriate.

Initial studies reported a 20- to 45-fold risk of thromboembolic events compared with cisgender controls, however these studies failed to control for tobacco use[36] and involved the use of high doses of oral ethinyl estradiol.[37] Ethinyl estradiol is a synthetic estrogen used in combination contraception preparations with a significant VTE risk.

The 17-β estradiol is currently the most commonly used estrogen in feminizing hormone regimens today and is chemically as well as biologically indistinguishable from endogenous ovarian estrogen. It may be administered as an oral/sublingual tablet, transdermal patch, or intramuscular/subcutaneous injection. Conjugated and synthetic estrogens use cannot be monitored serologically and confer no benefits over 17-β estradiol. Combined with their VTE risks, they are rarely used today when obtained through a physician.[18] The route of estradiol administration plays a described role on VTE risk.[38] The impact of estradiol on clotting factor synthesis is enhanced during first-pass metabolism.[39] Transdermal delivery of 17-β estradiol has been associated with a reduction in this risk.[40] Ideally, F-GAHT regimens include transdermal or IM estradiol formulations to address this concern.[41] Unfortunately, oral formulations of 17-β estradiol appear to be the most frequently prescribed in the United States due to cost and insurance limitations.[42]

Much of the rationale for perioperative estradiol discontinuation comes from a landmark study[39] noted that the following cessation of oral ethinyl estradiol a rebound in fibrinogen and antithrombin III concentrations were seen at 2 to 6 weeks. The authors postulated that surgery should be undertaken at least 4 weeks following cessation of oral ethinyl estradiol, at which stage fibrinogen is low, antithrombin III is high, and factor X has returned to baseline. This and subsequent studies evaluating the perioperative risk of estrogen were largely based on high doses of oral ethinyl estradiol. Furthermore, many of these studies were performed before the introduction of routine VTE prophylaxis and may not be applicable today. A recent meta-analysis review[43] of modern and historical feminizing GAHT regimens concluded that to date, there are no data to demonstrate the benefit of discontinuing estrogen-containing hormone regimes before major gender-affirming surgeries. The authors contend that for most young, healthy transgender women, there is little risk of VTE with continuation of perioperative hormone therapy, whereas older patients or those with additional risk factors should be considered on a individual basis.

Given the lack of randomized, controlled studies, many surgeons and societies, based largely on expert opinion recommend holding F-GAHT, in particular estrogens, for 2 to 6 weeks before and 3 to 4 weeks after "major" surgical procedures under general anesthesia.[44–49] Numerous professional societies have looked at perioperative VTE management in patients on F-GATH including the American Society of Plastic Surgeons, who in their VTE Task Force[50] published in 2012, recommended discontinuation of F-GAHT for all inpatient ("major") procedures under general anesthesia and for elective procedures in patients with Caprini scores ≥ 7. Other societies, including the American Association of Plastic Surgeons in 2016[51] and the European Society of Anaesthesiology in 2007,[52] recommend using the Caprini risk stratification to guide decision-making with less of a universal blanket policy regarding hormone therapy. The American College of Obstetricians and Gynecologists in 2018[53] recommended against routine preoperative discontinuation of hormone therapy and instead taking into consideration the risk of holding treatment as part of the overall calculus in those who may be at increased VTE risk. Perioperative discontinuation of estradiol may result in side effects that can have a significant mental and physical impact on quality of life, body image, and sexual function.[54] Two or six weeks after estradiol is stopped, virilization with testosterone occurs and serum estradiol concentrations may plummet to near the male reference range.[55] This risks preoperative rebound dysphoria with potential exacerbation of anxiety, depression, substance abuse, and suicidal ideation as well as physical effects.[56] This impact may result in perioperative harm and nonsurgical postoperative complications. According to Nolan and colleagues,[57] there is insufficient evidence to support routine discontinuation of estradiol therapy in the perioperative period. In all cases, it is recommended that patients complete a 2005 Caprini risk factor assessment (or equivalent) to stratify patients' VTE risk based on their individual risk factors and then apply the recommended mitigation strategies including early ambulation, mechanical prophylaxis, and chemoprophylaxis where appropriate. A risk factor common in the transgender population is the frequency in which they travel long distances to assess surgical care. The role of this specific risk factor on the overall calculus of perioperative F-GAHT cessation versus continuation is an area which needs to be investigated.

Although many of the negative effects of feminizing and masculinizing hormone therapies have been described, few studies have looked into how these effects specifically impact perioperative management. On such example is the changes in blood pressure found after initiating hormone therapy. A recent European Network for the Investigation of Gender Incongruence was the largest study ($n = 430$) that assessed blood pressure before and after initiating GAHT. In contrast to earlier smaller studies, it found that GAHT did not significantly change blood pressure in a clinically significant way.[58,59] Other potential issues which could impact the perioperative period include testosterone induced erythrocytosis, which has been reported in one in 4-to-6 transgender male depending on the formulation of testosterone.[60,61] The largest increase in hematocrit is typically observed within the first year. A reasonable first step in the care for transgender men with erythrocytosis while on testosterone is to advise smokers to quit, switch to a transdermal administration route if not already used, and address suboptimal BMI when present. There are data showing that as a whole the transgender population has a greater risk for cardiovascular disease with relatively high rates of undiagnosed and untreated comorbidities, such as hypertension and dyslipidemia, even before initiation of GAHT. The authors did not note how risk factors changed after GAHT.[62] A thorough preoperative cardiovascular risk assessment in transgender men is advisable.

Acne is a common adverse event with all testosterone formulations available today. Isotretinoin is being prescribed more frequently for refractory cases. Historically, recommendations were to wait 6 to 12 months after completion of isotretinoin therapy before considering elective surgical procedures on the head and neck. Although early reports suggested that isotretinoin use would impair wound healing, recent prospective clinical studies have not found an increased incidence of facial scarring in patients using isotretinoin in the perioperative period.[63]

Finally, individuals on GAHT, especially M-GAHT, have been noted to have modest increases in liver transaminases (ALT and AST concentrations) following testosterone initiation without clear clinical significance of the observed association.[64] Although seen, feminizing GAHT is less likely to induce appreciable changes in liver enzyme levels. Routine preoperative liver function testing is probably not necessary in patients on GAHT unless clinically indicated for other reasons.

SUMMARY

Hormone therapy is present in nearly every individual undergoing gender-affirming surgical procedures of the head and neck. Head and neck surgeons need to be aware of the role, expectations, limitations, and negative effects of GAHT could have in the perioperative period. The limited availability of randomized controlled data sets guiding evidence-based perioperative hormone therapy management in transgender individuals has resulted in guidelines based primarily on expert opinion or limited observational studies. Many of these guidelines fail to take into consideration the risks of perioperative GAHT discontinuation.

CLINICS CARE POINTS

- Patients should be fully living the life of the affirmed gender for at least 12 continuous months on appropriate gender-affirming hormone therapy (GAHT) before considering irreversible gender-affirming surgical procedures of the face, neck, and voice.
- Patients should be given ample time on GAHT to realize reasonably expected changes in secondary sex characteristics.
- Careful postoperative planning is essential as many patients receive surgical care hundreds or thousands of miles from home with suboptimal support systems.
- The perioperative risks of continuing GAHT should also be weighed against the risks of hormone discontinuation.

DISCLOSURE

No financial or conflicts of interest to disclose.

REFERENCES

1. Meerwijk EL, Sevelius JM. Transgender population size in the united states: a meta- regression of population-based probability samples. Am J Public Health 2017;107(2):e1–8.
2. Available at: https://www1.nyc.gov/assets/cchr/downloads/pdf/publications/GenderID_Card2015.pdf. Accessed February 14, 2022.
3. Leinung MC, Joseph J. Changing demographics in transgender individuals seeking hormonal therapy: are trans women more common than trans men? Transgend Health 2020;5(4):241–5.
4. Nolan IT, Kuhner CJ, Dy GW. Demographic and temporal trends in transgender identities and gender confirming surgery. Transl Androl Urol 2019;8(3):184–90.
5. Bradley SJ, Blanchard R, Coates S, et al. Interim report of the DSM-IV subcommittee on gender identity disorders. Arch Sex Behav 1991;20(4):333–43.
6. Available at: https://www.psychiatry.org/File%20Library/Psychiatrists/Practice/DSM/APA_DSM-5-Gender- Dysphoria.pdf. Accessed February 14, 2022.
7. James SE, Herman JL, Rankin S, et al. The report of the 2015 U.S. transgender survey. Washington, DC: National Center for Transgender Equality; 2016.
8. Feldman JL, Luhur WE, Herman JL, et al. Health and health care access in the US transgender population health (TransPop) survey. Andrology 2021;9(6):1707–18.
9. Zaliznyak M, Yuan N, Bresee C, et al. How early in life do transgender adults begin to experience gender dysphoria? why this matters for patients, providers, and for our healthcare system. Sex Med 2021;9(6):100448.
10. Kuper LE, Stewart S, Preston S, et al. Body dissatisfaction and mental health outcomes of youth on gender-affirming hormone therapy. Pediatrics 2020;145(4): e20193006.
11. O'Connell MA, Nguyen TP, Ahler A, et al. Approach to the patient: pharmacological management of trans and gender diverse adolescents. J Clin Endocrinol Metab 2021. https://doi.org/10.1210/clinem/dgab634.
12. van der Loos MA, Hellinga I, Vlot MC, et al. Development of hip bone geometry during gender-affirming hormone therapy in transgender adolescents resembles that of the experienced gender when pubertal suspension is started in early puberty. J Bone Miner Res 2021;36(5):931–41.

13. Weinand JD, Safer JD. Hormone therapy in transgender adults is safe with provider supervision; A review of hormone therapy sequelae for transgender individuals. J Clin Transl Endocrinol 2015;2(2):55–60.
14. Foster Skewis L, Bretherton I, Leemaqz SY, et al. Short-term effects of gender-affirming hormone therapy on dysphoria and quality of life in transgender individuals: a prospective controlled study. Front Endocrinol (Lausanne) 2021;12: 717766.
15. Meyer G, Mayer M, Mondorf A, et al. Safety and rapid efficacy of guideline-based gender-affirming hormone therapy: an analysis of 388 individuals diagnosed with gender dysphoria. Eur J Endocrinol 2020;182(2):149–56.
16. Coleman E, Bockting W, Botzer M, et al. Standards of care for the health of transsexual, transgender, and gender-nonconforming people, version 7. Int J Transgend 2011;13:165.
17. Fraser L, Knudson G. Past and future challenges associated with standards of care for gender transitioning clients. Psychiatr Clin North Am 2017;40(1):15–27.
18. Hembree WC, Cohen-Kettenis PT, Gooren L, et al. Endocrine treatment of gender- dysphoric/gender-incongruent persons: an endocrine society clinical practice guideline. J Clin Endocrinol Metab 2017;102(11):3869–903.
19. Dahlen S, Connolly D, Arif I, et al. International clinical practice guidelines for gender minority/trans people: systematic review and quality assessment. BMJ Open 2021;11(4):e048943.
20. Telfer MM, Tollit MA, Pace CC, et al. Australian standards of care and treatment guidelines for transgender and gender diverse children and adolescents. Med J Aust 2018;209(3):132–6. https://doi.org/10.5694/mja17.01044.
21. Chen S, Loshak H. 2020. Cited in: Ovid MEDLINE(R) Epub Ahead of Print at Available at. http://ovidsp.ovid.com/ovidweb.cgi?T=JS&PAGE=reference&D= medp&NEWS=N&AN=33112530. Accessed December 06, 2021.
22. Inwards-Breland DJ, Karrington B, Sequeira GM. Access to care for transgender and nonbinary youth: ponder this, innumerable barriers exist. JAMA Pediatr 2021; 175(11):1112–4.
23. Haupt C, Henke M, Kutschmar A, et al. Antiandrogen or estradiol treatment or both during hormone therapy in transitioning transgender women. Cochrane Database Syst Rev 2020;11:CD013138.
24. Greene DN, Schmidt RL, Winston McPherson G, et al. Reproductive endocrinology reference intervals for transgender women on stable hormone therapy. J Appl Lab Med 2021;6(1):15–26.
25. Prior JC. Progesterone is important for transgender women's therapy-applying evidence for the benefits of progesterone in ciswomen. J Clin Endocrinol Metab 2019;104(4):1181–6.
26. Prince JCJ, Safer JD. Endocrine treatment of transgender individuals: current guidelines and strategies. Expert Rev Endocrinol Metab 2020;15(6):395–403.
27. Harper J, O'Donnell E, Sorouri Khorashad B, et al. How does hormone transition in transgender women change body composition, muscle strength and haemoglobin? Systematic review with a focus on the implications for sport participation. BJSM Online 2021;55(15):865–72.
28. Silva ED, Fighera TM, Allgayer RM, et al. Physical and sociodemographic features associated with quality of life among transgender women and men using gender-affirming hormone therapy. Front Psychiatr 2021;12:621075.
29. Masumori N, Baba T, Abe T, et al. What is the most anticipated change induced by treatment using gender-affirming hormones in individuals with gender incongruence? Int J Urol 2021;28(5):526–9.

30. Aschenbrenner DS. First Oral Testosterone Product Now Available. Am J Nurs 2019;119(8):22–3.
31. Unger CA. Hormone therapy for transgender patients. Transl Androl Urol 2016; 5(6):877–84.
32. Hodges-Simeon CR, Grail GPO, Albert G, et al. Testosterone therapy masculinizes speech and gender presentation in transgender men. Sci Rep 2021;11(1): 3494.
33. Morrison SD, Vyas KS, Motakef S, et al. Facial feminization: systematic review of the literature. Plast Reconstr Surg 2016;137(6):1759–70.
34. Hontscharuk R, Alba B, Manno C, et al. Perioperative transgender hormone management: avoiding venous thromboembolism and other complications. Plast Reconstr Surg 2021;147(4):1008–17.
35. Kotamarti VS, Greige N, Heiman AJ, et al. Risk for venous thromboembolism in transgender patients undergoing cross-sex hormone treatment: a systematic review. J Sex Med 2021;18(7):1280–91.
36. Asscheman H, Gooren LJ, Eklund PL. Mortality and morbidity in transsexual patients with cross-gender hormone treatment. Metabolism 1989;38(9):869–73.
37. van Kesteren PJ, Asscheman H, Megens JA, et al. Mortality and morbidity in transsexual subjects treated with cross-sex hormones. Clin Endocrinol (Oxf) 1997;47(3):337–42.
38. Scarabin PY, Oger E, Plu-Bureau G. EStrogen and THromboEmbolism Risk Study Group. Differential association of oral and transdermal oestrogen-replacement therapy with venous thromboembolism risk. Lancet 2003;362(9382):428–32.
39. Robinson GE, Burren T, Mackie IJ, et al. Changes in haemostasis after stopping the combined contraceptive pill: implications for major surgery. BMJ 1991; 302(6771):269–71.
40. Price TM, Blauer KL, Hansen M, et al. Single-dose pharmacokinetics of sublingual versus oral administration of micronized 17 beta-estradiol. Obstet Gynecol 1997;89(3):340–5.
41. Gooren LJ, T'Sjoen G. Endocrine treatment of aging transgender people. Rev Endocr Metab Disord 2018;19(3):253–62.
42. Solotke MT, Liu P, Dhruva SS, et al. Medicare prescription drug plan coverage of hormone therapies used by transgender individuals. LGBT health 2020;7(3): 137–45.
43. Zucker R, Reisman T, Safer JD. Minimizing venous thromboembolism in feminizing hormone therapy: applying lessons from cisgender women and previous data. Endocr Pract 2021;27(6):621–5.
44. Reed HM. Aesthetic and functional male to female genital and perineal surgery: feminizing vaginoplasty. Semin Plast Surg 2011;25(2):163–74.
45. Buncamper ME, van der Sluis WB, van der Pas RSD, et al. Surgical outcome after penile inversion vaginoplasty: a retrospective study of 475 transgender women. Plast Reconstr Surg 2016;138(5):999–1007.
46. Goddard JC, Vickery RM, Qureshi A, et al. Feminizing genitoplasty in adult transsexuals: early and long-term surgical results. BJU Int 2007;100(3):607–13.
47. Asscheman H, T'Sjoen G, Lemaire A, et al. Venous thrombo-embolism as a complication of cross-sex hormone treatment of male-to-female transsexual subjects: a review. Andrologia 2014;46(7):791–5.
48. Shatzel JJ, Connelly KJ, DeLoughery TG. Thrombotic issues in transgender medicine: a review. Am J Hematol 2017;92(2):204–8.
49. Godano A, Maggi M, Jannini E, et al. SIAMS-ONIG Consensus on hormonal treatment in gender identity disorders. J Endocrinol Invest 2009;32(10):857–64.

50. Murphy RX Jr, Alderman A, Gutowski K, et al. Evidence-based practices for thromboembolism prevention: summary of the ASPS Venous Thromboembolism Task Force Report. Plast Reconstr Surg 2012;130(1):168e–75e.
51. Pannucci CJ, MacDonald JK, Ariyan S, et al. Benefits and Risks of Prophylaxis for Deep Venous Thrombosis and Pulmonary Embolus in Plastic Surgery: A Systematic Review and Meta-Analysis of Controlled Trials and Consensus Conference. Plast Reconstr Surg 2016;137(2):709–30.
52. Afshari A, Ageno W, Ahmed A, et al, ESA VTE Guidelines Task Force. European guidelines on perioperative venous thromboembolism prophylaxis: Executive summary. Eur J Anaesthesiol 2018;35:77–83.
53. ACOG Committee Opinion No. 750: perioperative pathways: enhanced recovery after surgery. Obstet Gynecol 2018;132(3):e120–30.
54. Lawrence AA. Patient-reported complications and functional outcomes of male-to-female sex reassignment surgery. Arch Sex Behav 2006;35(6):717–27.
55. Schneider F, Neuhaus N, Wistuba J, et al. Testicular functions and clinical characterization of patients with gender dysphoria (GD) undergoing sex reassignment surgery (SRS). J Sex Med 2015;12(11):2190–200.
56. Tollinche LE, Walters CB, Radix A, et al. The Perioperative Care of the Transgender Patient. Anesth Analg 2018;127(2):359–66.
57. Nolan BJ, Cheung AS. Estradiol Therapy in the Perioperative Period: Implications for Transgender People Undergoing Feminizing Hormone Therapy. Yale J Biol Med 2020;93(4):539–48. Cited in: Ovid MEDLINE(R) at Available at: http://ovidsp.ovid.com/ovidweb.cgi?T=JS&PAGE=reference&D=medl&NEWS=N&AN=33005118. Accessed December 04, 2021.
58. van Velzen DM, Paldino A, Klaver M, et al. Cardiometabolic effects of testosterone in transmen and estrogen plus cyproterone acetate in transwomen. J Clin Endocrinol Metab 2019;104(6):1937–47. https://doi.org/10.1210/jc.2018-02138.
59. Connelly PJ, Clark A, Touyz RM, et al. Transgender adults, gender-affirming hormone therapy and blood pressure: a systematic review. J Hypertens 2021;39(2):223–30.
60. Nolan BJ, Leemaqz SY, Ooi O, et al. Prevalence of polycythaemia with different formulations of testosterone therapy in transmasculine individuals. Intern Med J 2021;51(6):873–8.
61. Madsen MC, van Dijk D, Wiepjes CM, et al. Erythrocytosis in a large cohort of trans men using testosterone: a long-term follow-up study on prevalence, determinants, and exposure years. J Clin Endocrinol Metab 2021;106(6):1710–7.
62. Denby KJ, Cho L, Toljan K, et al. Assessment of cardiovascular risk in transgender patients presenting for gender-affirming care. Am J Med 2021;134(8):1002–8.
63. Gulati RD, Faraci N, Butts SC. Neonatal ear molding. Laryngoscope 2021;131(2):E423–7.
64. Hashemi L, Zhang Q, Getahun D, et al. Longitudinal changes in liver enzyme levels among transgender people receiving gender affirming hormone therapy. J Sex Med 2021;18(9):1662–75.

Modern Responses to Traditional Pitfalls in Gender Affirming Behavioral Voice Modification

Amelia Zheanna Huff, BA

KEYWORDS

- Gender-affirming voice modification • Transgender voice • Vocal resonance
- Vocal gender • Voice learning • Voice therapy • Voice dysphoria

KEY POINTS

- Institutional support is built around outside observer-developed practices, which risk delaying the effectiveness and rate of progress in gender voice modification.
- Ear training is essential for clinicians and voice learners.
- Clinicians should be aware of limitations in surgical intervention in order to better develop multidisciplinary solutions for gender and sex modification of the voice.
- Resonance is frequently mischaracterized, and current clinical standards of resonance training need improvement.

Audio content accompanies this article at http://www.oto.theclinics.com.

INTRODUCTION

Gender-affirming behavioral voice modification (GABVM) is a form of voice habilitation in which a voice user works to gain control over their voice to effectively alter the gender and sex perception of their speech, singing, or reflexive sounds. This is done to alleviate gender dysphoria or better align the gender expression of their communication to their gender identity. Traditionally, this practice has been guided and studied primarily by cisgender speech language pathologists (SLPs) who do not actively modify their voice, or behaviorally normalize a new vocal presentation. Meanwhile, this process is lived by transgender and gender-diverse people in their daily lives. As such, clinicians act as outside observers, yet drive the institutions, research, and standards of care. This landscape encourages oversight of basic voice learning fundamentals, such as effective practice strategies, direct modeling of target

TransVoiceLessons and Internal Bioacoustics LLC, 5815 SE Rhone Street, Portland, OR 97206, USA
E-mail address: ZheaEroseMusic@gmail.com

Otolaryngol Clin N Am 55 (2022) 727–738
https://doi.org/10.1016/j.otc.2022.05.001
0030-6665/22/© 2022 Elsevier Inc. All rights reserved.

actions, and auditory dominant learning. Oversights of such basic voice learning fundamentals diminish the quality of care for trans people if unaddressed by the clinical community. The goal of this article is to raise awareness about many of these structural and technical pitfalls in the current landscape and standard of care maintained by clinicians and to offer strategies for improvement.[1-8]

It is imperative to advance new strategies, methods, and solutions to provide an increasingly effective framework for hearing, interacting, and ultimately controlling the vocal acoustic markers which express sex and gender. Current clinical practice primarily consists of basic pitch training, usage of semioccluded vocal tract exercises, a lack of clear guidance on resonance control, clinicians with little experience on permanently altering their own voices, and an overemphasis on proprioceptive dominant learning rather than auditory focused learning. Although some of these tools are certainly useful, improvements can be made to better meet clients' needs.

For example, standard pitch training can be improved by also training the ear to hear source spectral excitement as perceptual "vocal weight" alongside pitch. Weight tends to work antagonistically against pitch which often impairs the effectiveness of pitch training alone. This relationship is not discussed in standard clinical practice yet acts as a crucial backbone in vocal fundamentals. In addition, it should be standard that clinicians either have direct experience in modifying their own voice or have received instruction by someone with experience in voice modification. Perhaps the most important need is a shift toward greater emphasis on auditory targets acquired through ear training and behavioral modeling. An auditory target transmits the blueprint for control of the voice. Therefore, to efficiently teach something like resonance modification, curated sound patterns must be learned, which correspond to the desired vocal tract movements. These fundamental pitfalls and possible solutions are discussed herein in the hopes of encouraging growth for clinicians, clinical practice, and those in need of effective gender-affirming care.

UNDERSTANDING THE FUNDAMENTALS

Differences between average masculine and feminine voices are created by a complex interaction between physiologic and sociocultural components, which inseparably fuse together to form a speaker's timbre and style. Physiologically, testosterone exposure causes growth to the vocal folds and vocal tract. Average male vocal folds are roughly 25% longer and 20% thicker than average female vocal folds, whereas the total pharyngeal volume sees a 70% increase during pubertal exposure to testosterone. Many other nuanced morphometric differences can be seen, such as oral cavity volume, vocal tract length, and lung capacity. Not all differences in vocal sex and gender perception are purely the result of morphologic differences from sexual development. By the age of 4 years, there are already noticeable acoustic differences between the vowel formants in voices of young boys and girls, and by the age of 6 years, there are measurable differences in mean fundamental frequency despite no significant physiologic differences observed in the vocal tract. This implicates sociocultural factors, which mold behavior across gendered lines. In this way, for the purpose of this article, it may be useful to make a distinction between *gendered* and *sexed* aspects of voice, whereby gendered refers to primarily sociocultural patterns and sexed refers to acoustic markers from morphologic differences despite their inextricable entanglement. Sex modifications tend to carry an auditory implication of a different underlying "body," whereas gender modifications carry an implication of a different social or environmental history.

With both gender and sex components to voice, transgender and gender nonconforming individuals may find incongruity between their internal identity and their outward vocal presentation. Thus, voice dysphoria is the manifestation of gender dysphoria as it relates to the sound, sensation, and communication effect of one's own speaking voice. Vocal dysphoria can be extremely debilitating and greatly reduce quality of life. Incongruence between internal identity and patterns of vocal expression can cause social, psychological, and physical harm. The experience of vocal dysphoria is diverse and unique to each individual, which requires the clinician to deeply listen to each individual's needs.

Although not all trans people suffer from voice dysphoria and not all people who experience voice dysphoria identify as trans, it is crucial to have effective systems to care for and reduce harm for those who need to change their voice. In these cases, clinicians need to inquire and carefully listen to the individual's vocal needs and goals, as each case will be different. Vocal health, fitness, function, and proficiency should be assessed in order to provide a safe and efficient pathway forward. Regardless of the specific target goal, an effective approach will almost always include substantial ear training, motor skills training, and behavioral training. Realignment of outward communication style toward the desired goal of the speaker and behavioral normalization of that goal should mirror the process of how babies and children are guided through the acquisition of speech. Voice learning in humans occurs through the acquisition of auditory templates modeled and exaggerated by caregivers. Because of this, the use of ear training with accurate behavioral modeling is essential in treating voice dysphoria. Ear training consists of repeated exposure to auditory targets in order to internalize them clearly so one can mentally imagine, mentally control, improve identification, and develop the ability to detect proximity to the target sounds. Ear training is a fundamental skill in music learning and basic speech acquisition, yet it tends to be absent in clinical practice of GABVM. Clinicians must be able to actively demonstrate the vocal modifications they are leading their students to imitate in order for adequate auditory learning to take root. If a clinician cannot clearly demonstrate the shift in sound they want the client to learn, it is equivalent to trying to teach a baby a language they do not speak. This is the most serious limitation of the observer-directed clinical approach. One must be able to *do* the action to properly nourish the client's ear to ensure success.

ON INSTITUTIONAL AND OBSERVER ENTANGLEMENT

The origin of these issues comes from the entanglement between observer-generated methodology and institutional authority. Although institutional systems dedicated to transgender individuals have progressed compared to a few decades ago, there is more work to be done. The traditional model for gender-affirming voice modification has been primarily developed and maintained by cisgender SLPs. The current standards of care as recommended by the World Professional Association of Transgender Health anchors SLPs as the "primary providers of service" while describing all non-SLPs as an "adjunct role." The American Speech-Language-Hearing Association also positions SLPs as the "central role" in gender-affirming voice modification. Two primary educational texts in the field, *Voice and Communication Therapy for the Transgender/Gender Diverse Client: A Comprehensive Clinical Guide* by Hirsch and Adler and *The Voice Book for Trans and Non-Binary People: A Practical Guide to Creating and Sustaining Authentic Voice and Communication* by Mills and Stoneham,[10] are both written by cisgender SLPs in which only direct accounts of the skill and process of voice modification are given through anecdotal citations of trans voices.[19] Furthermore, on Liz Jackson's *Trans Affirming Teacher Referral List*, there are currently 135 respondents.[11] Of those, only 12 identify as transgender and only 12 identify as

nonbinary, which means 82% are cisgender. When observers, rather than participants, are driving the conversation and training other clinicians in methodology, the
stage is set for oversights. These gaps in understanding are discussed in this article.

Speech pathologists are skilled experts in voice *rehabilitation*. GABVM is voice
habituation and *habilitation*, as there is nothing inherently disordered or damaged
about a voice seeking to feminize, masculinize, or androgynize. Pathologizing and
treating impaired voices is not adequate training for GABVM. The education that general speech pathologists undergo does not focus on ear training, voice control, personal application of vocal motor skills in a gender-modifying way, or the lived
experience of normalizing a new voice quality. Vocal behavior is transmitted aurally,
not textually. Vocal motor skills stem from first having auditory templates to guide action. There are too many nonlinearities and auditory-motor nuances to have a complete understanding of the topic from reading.

Institutional authority imbues a clinician with inherent credibility and insurance
support. The title of licensed SLP instills confidence in many trans individuals. Insurance benefits for SLP care providers create an environment that drives the trans
population toward SLPs for care. However, although qualified SLPs certainly exist,
the certification and title of SLP are not synonymous with being proficient in this
practice. This is especially problematic if a client does not achieve the goals they
want. The disappointment is enhanced by feeling as if the official and medically
recognized resources did not work for them. This is despite these "medically recognized" sources often having little direct experience in modifying the gender of their
own voices. The last point of concern surrounding the structure of institutionalization
in this field involves empirical testing around the effectiveness of models that exist
outside of the SLP community. Conducting or contributing to the body of academic
research is made more difficult by barriers of funding, networking, and lack of credibility carried by operating outside of the academic environment. Clinicians should
be aware of these power dynamics in the institutional structures and how observer
bias may influence their practice. This imbalance in power can be resolved by
greater inclusion and amplification of transgender and gender-diverse voices in
the field, allocation of resources by the institutional network to those with lived experience but no systemic backing to do proper research, and redefining what adequate
training means in the clinical space.

EAR TRAINING IS ESSENTIAL AND ESSENTIALLY MISSING

Ear training is the process of exposing the ear to patterns of sound in order to develop
greater aural awareness, recognition, and comprehension. Ear training is absolutely
essential to voice learning. Humans are shown to learn voice through exposure to
acoustic models, which become auditory templates, which is then compared with
vocal action.[9–13] This allows the user to have meta-auditive ability, and attempts toward vocalization can be assessed to generate self-feedback. Self-feedback is crucial
to long-term success in GAVBM. The ability to hear creates a path forward for action
reflection. Ear training should not be treated as supplementary; it is the *primary tool* in
which vocal learning progression is built by. However, discussions of ear training are
missing from the main pieces of literature, which have guided GABVM in speech language pathology practice. Most textbooks and journal articles discussing sex and
gender modification in speech are devoid of sound files, auditory targets, and methodology for training the ear.

The lack of ear training for both clinicians and clients in the current field begs to be
addressed. This oversight is an example of how outsider observers who have not lived

the experience they are trying to teach can overlook very simple and necessary aspects of the process. An individual who does not have to modify their own voice may not see the need for auditory templates; however, this is crucial in the modification of voice.

There are several ways to train the ear. Ear training can be divided into active or passive and immersive or nonimmersive, and all combinations have value and application. **Fig. 1** displays 4 types.

Active types of ear training involve listening to specific sounds and consciously trying to listen toward them, remember them, audiate them internally, imitate them, and reflect on them. During this process, it is very beneficial to have a student subjectively describe what the target sounds like, what it reminds them of, and to identify any associations they have to the sound. Passive ear training involves hearing the sound without consciously focusing on it. Nonimmersive ear training is acute exposure to target patterns, such as vocal demonstrations in a lecture or lesson or a short practice session. On the other hand, immersive forms of ear training involve sustained saturation of the ears in a target sound, such as listening to a long playlist of target voices throughout an entire day or practicing constantly throughout the day. A parallel can be made to language learning. Learning a new language in a classroom is nonimmersive. Traveling to a new country to learn a language is immersive. Immersive ear training is almost completely absent from the clinical discourse around gender-affirming voice modification. However, immersive forms of ear training enable listeners to acquire complex nuances, which are otherwise hard to distill as simple technique. Just as students of language will travel to a culture to immerse themselves in the sound of the language in order to pick up the nuances of the style, the same immersion process should be taken advantage of in GAVBM in order for an individual to pick up culturally and socially relevant patterns aligned with their goals. In language learning, stylistic elements, such as rhythm, pitch contour, and articulation, may sound awkward or "unnatural" even after a speaker can technically hold a conversation in their new language. The usage of immersion may assist toward learning nuances in communication style. The same process may be used in gender-affirming voice training by creating opportunities for immersion, such as long playlists of target sounds, daily habitual use of a target voice, or the creation of voice learning communities to encourage greater emphasis on aural exposure.

Auditory exposure is fundamental to voice learning. The way in which sounds are modeled to an individual learning makes a significant difference. As such, a clinician teaching vocal gender modification should be able to strongly modify the gender of their own speech in order to give an auditory template and an effective behavioral map to the client. In this case, a non-androgen-exposed voice simply modeling itself for an androgenized voice to follow, such as in the case of an average ciswoman teaching an average transwoman, is *not* the same transmitted blueprint as an androgenized voice modeling feminization for another androgenized voice to follow. Sound is the map for vocal action. This asymmetry can be mitigated, but it requires the clinician to have the ability to feminize or masculinize their voice further than their default.

Active Immersion	Passive Immersion
Active Non Immersion	Passive Non Immersion

Fig. 1. Primary forms of ear training.

LIMITS OF SURGICAL MODIFICATION

Surgical modifications to feminize or masculinize the vocal physiology, such as forms of glottoplasty, pharyngeal plication, thyrohyoid elevation, or cricothyroid approximation, do not address behavioral elements that are acquired through socialization. As discussed, there are noticeable acoustic differences between the vowel formants and mean fundamental frequency in the voices of young boys and girls despite no significant physiologic differences observed in the vocal tract.

These socially transmitted, non-physiology-based differences cannot be accounted for via modification of physical structures. Instead, these differences show up as dynamic learned movements.[14] These elements incapable of surgical modification are not the physical *structure* of the vocal tract and vocal folds but instead the active *movement* of these physical components to generate speech. Clinicians should be aware of the dynamic, cultural, and performative aspects of communication and inform patients of what voice surgery has the possibility to alter and what it does not.

Current surgical intervention, such as glottoplasty or cricothyroid approximation, attempts to work by elevating fundamental pitch and reducing vocal weight of the speaker through reduction of vocal fold mass. Surgical approaches like this are the most common, but they do not address resonance, pitch contour, articulation, and other important aspects in GABVM. More recently, surgical methods for altering resonance, such as pharyngeal plication, are expanding, but these are still quite limited in their effect. Surgery, unfortunately, cannot give vocal control.

It is therefore necessary that implementation of basic ear training and auditory immersion be used alongside surgery to yield better outcomes. Strategies such as providing a lengthy playlist full of diverse voices in the direction of the patient's goal can be used in addition to surgery. Patients should be encouraged to listen to and mimic along with auditory clips to improve the outcomes of vocal surgery. There is fertile ground for implementing basic auditory learning by immersion into the surgical recovery process to achieve better outcomes, even in situations where the patient chooses not to behaviorally train the voice.

RESONANCE: A CLINICAL BLIND SPOT

The manipulation and awareness of vocal resonance are a core component to effective gender and sex modification. One of the gaps between teaching and practice in GABVM is evident in the way vocal resonance techniques are discussed and taught. There is a gap between research on vocal sex dimorphism and how to apply that information to achieve behavioral sex and gender modification. An accurate, efficient, and impactful auditory framework for guiding voices to control resonance in a sex-modulating way is necessary to achieve best results. The traditional model is dominated by somatic sensory descriptions, such as descriptions of "moving vibrations out of the chest,"[15] highly subjective behavior prompts like "placing sound forward,"[9,15-20] and other difficult-to-reliably-replicate tricks disconnected from auditory patterns corresponding to the acoustic effect of sex difference in the vocal tract.[20] Instead, careful auditory targets, which act as maps for effective resonance modification, should be instituted, which is described in later discussion.

The vocal tract acts as a complex resonance chamber, which attenuates and modulates sound passing through it. Depending on the size, shape, material properties, and other nuances of the vocal tract, a unique spectral filter profile emerges, creating a distinct coloration of the sound.[21] Human vocal tracts are complex, elastic, and nonuniform resonators composed of numerous sections, which relate nonlinearly, forming multiple resonances capable of a diverse array of relationships. The audible and measurable effect of these resonances acting on the sound can be heard and measured. These measurable and perceivable spectral peaks are called formants.[22]

Perceptual vowel quality is strongly determined by the position, strength, and relativity between formants.[23] **Fig. 2** (Audio 2) shows several spectral filter patterns of formant activity that correspond to vowel identity modeled after 3 basic vowels, /i/, /a/, and/ae/. These spectral illustrations are created by imprinting a filter pattern onto white noise and will be referred to as formant-filter patterns. These visualize general movements of resonance, which voices are capable of re-creating. Audio files of these patterns can be heard from the attached audio with both noise and harmonic prefilter sources. Perceptual vowel quality can be interpreted aurally and as an expression of the resonance, and thus give information about the vocal tract's shape, size, and behavior Audios 1–5.

Fig. 3 (Audio 4) shows 2 examples of shifts in formant-filter. In these examples, the sound is modulated to form 2 distinct shifts vowel identities, /i/ to /ae/ and /i/ to /ʌ/. Formant shifts, such as this that cause perceptual phonemic identity to change, tend to have little influence over gender or sex perception. Patterns like these will be referred to as shifts in *perceptual vowel identity* and do not strongly influence the perception of vocal sex. These patterns permeate most of an individual's formant behavior during speech and form the background of resonance activity that consonant sounds punctuate. An audio file of these patterns synthesized and behaviorally performed is attached.

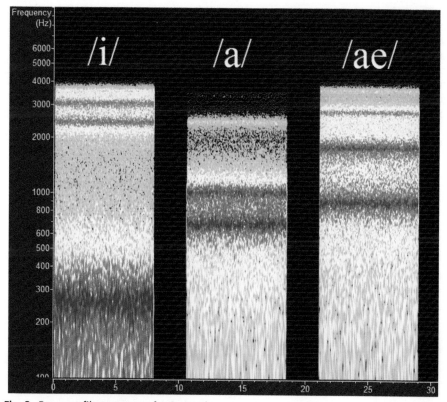

Fig. 2. Formant-filter patterns for 3 vowels.

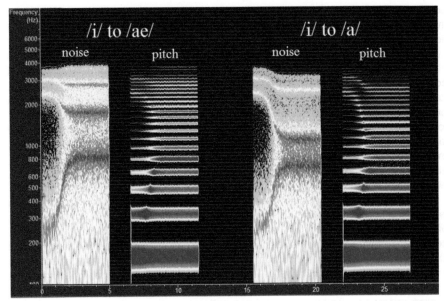

Fig. 3. Examples of perceptual vowel identity shifting.

Fig. 4 (Audio 5) shows a different pattern of formant-filter shifting. In these examples, the sound is modulated to preserve one single perceptual vowel identity but with shifts in *perceptual vowel size*. Perceptual size has profound impact on gender and sex perception. These types of auditory shifts correspond with a visible scaling pattern in the formant-filter. This scaling pattern is achieved by a complex transformation of the vocal tract dimensions, which mirrors changes androgen exposure induces (or the reversal of androgen exposure). Formant scaling patterns are profoundly powerful in gender and sex modification of voice.

Perceptual size as a result of formant scaling forms a reliable basis for teaching the modification of resonance to clients. This shift is a pattern capable of being

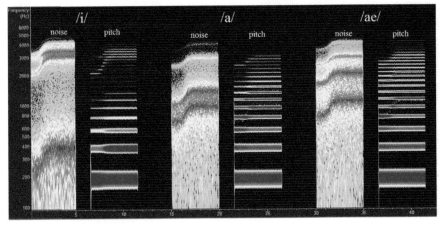

Fig. 4. Formant-filter patterns of vowel scaling.

behaviorally demonstrated, digitally modeled, quantified, and even used as a predictive tool to derive the transformative path of a vowel undergoing gender and sex modification. **Fig. 5** illustrates 2 more of these scaling shifts to core vowel identities, /i/, and /ʌ/. Audio files are a more detailed behavioral demonstration of size modification.

Clinicians teaching gender-affirming voice modification should be able to hear and control this pattern of resonance modification across all vowels and speech as a whole. The ability to audibly demonstrate a gender and sex modification of resonance provides the auditory template to the required physical movement the student needs to succeed in their goals. If seeking to mirror adult vocal learning with childhood vocal learning, it is essential for the instructor to exaggerate and demonstrate the entire movement of how to get to the target rather than just the final target by itself. Being able to fluidly model and speak these shifts to clients provides useful auditory templates to encourage the development of sex perception modulating actions.

Perceptual size functions effectively in the author's practice as a clear auditory pattern that clients can use to help accurately reduce or increase the size and shape of the vocal tract to meet their desired vocal goals. The goal should be to reduce the perceptual *size* of a target vowel without allowing the phonemic identity of the vowel to shift. When the vocal tract scales larger or smaller based on development sex differences, all vocal tract resonances shift together.[24] The corresponding effect is the preservation of a vowel's perceptual identity, whereas its perceptual size shifts. Vowel scaling patterns represent a distilled form of resonance modification shifting across a sexed continuum.

This method is absent in the techniques of resonance modification being taught in the current models. We see leading publications instead use subjective description of chest versus head resonance, /i/-ification of a vowel, and subjective descriptions of "moving the sound forward." Unfortunately, these all have problematic aspects. In the descriptions of chest versus head resonance, this is often used to describe how much "vibration" or intensity a voice user feels in their head or chest.[15] This is problematic because, observationally, the source spectral roll off[25] is the primary driver,

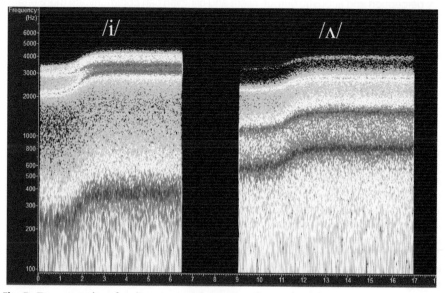

Fig. 5. Two examples of scaling a vowel from masculine to feminine.

which causes voice users to describe a sound experience as "in the chest" or "in the head." Source spectral roll off is an acoustic property illustrated by instruments that have a tendency to become buzzier and more metallic sounding as they increase in intensity. In voice, this quality is driven by a change in sound production. As such, it is not a *resonance* change because it is not a change in vocal tract structure. Rather, it is a shift in *sound production* primarily involving the vocal folds, which is currently being mislabeled as a resonance change in current clinical practice. This risks misleading students to modifications of source spectra rather than behavioral modifications of the vocal tract and leads to confusion surrounding how to hear resonance.

Another pedagogical pitfall of training resonance control can be seen in varying texts in which SLPs describe coaching students toward "/i/-ifying a vowel."[15,26] Essentially, this encourages the client speaking in a posture similar to the configuration, which generates the formant-filter pattern for /i/. However, this is quite problematic, as when we listen and analyze the resonance patterns of the /i/ vowel, we see a very low F1 and very high F2. Gender modification of resonance should manifest as movement of all primary formants in the same direction. When using an /i/-ifying technique, instead you will tend to see F1 lower or stay the same while F2 raises. With the /i/-ification of the voice, an instructor essentially encourages the client to have the same or more pharyngeal volume from their neutral /i/ vowel while encouraging a very small oral cavity. Reflecting on previous discussions of vocal tract size, this does not adequately address the total pharyngeal volume discrepancy between masculine and feminine vocal tracts.[27] Instead, it overexaggerates reduction of the oral cavity volume.

Last, there is a common somatic sensory approach whereby a client is instructed to "place the sound further forward."[15] Placement method has been used as the primary prompt for feminizing or masculinizing resonance in SLP work up to this point.[20] This approach is not based on an auditory phenomenon and does not teach the student to *hear* the influence of resonance on the voice. The experience of "placing" the sound is highly subjective and does not inherently correspond to spatial reduction patterns in the vocal tract for the most perceptual sex modulation.[26] By instead focusing on auditory perception and acoustic output, client and clinician can communicate more effectively and accurately.

REFLECTIONS

Vocal dysphoria profoundly impacts quality of life. Powerful GABVM instruction saves lives. Because the need is so great, clinicians should be called on to develop practical skill in voice modification in order to become active participants rather than active observers to better guide their clients. Proficiency in voice modification allows clinicians to demonstrate and model for students to quickly form auditory templates, which facilitate the necessary motor skills development. Currently, outside observers drive the institutions, trajectory of research, and standards of care. There are many factors discussed in this article that should be addressed to improve the quality of care. Ear training needs to become a central part of clinician training for those seeking to teach sex and gender modification of speech. Movement toward practical models focused on ear training and motor skills around acoustic signatures of vocal sex needs to take precedent. Awareness of surgical limitations may help surgeons develop more holistic strategies to achieve more satisfactory results and better manage patient's expectations around gender-affirming vocal surgery. Current clinical standards of resonance training need to be reworked to better serve the trans community. As an alternative, the author has proposed a model using perceptual size based on the auditory experience of a vocal tract expanding or shrinking in volume according to sexed averages and proportions. Moving forward, the author hopes to see adaptation around these aforementioned critical areas in order to better serve the needs of transgender and gender nonconforming individuals. By working together to dissolve boundaries between observers and participants, we can better improve the outcomes of GABVM to improve the lives of transgender and gender nonconforming people everywhere.

DISCLOSURE

The author has no financial conflicts of interest other than being an educator in the field.

SUPPLEMENTARY DATA

Supplementary data related to this article can be found online at https://doi.org/10.1016/j.otc.2022.05.001.

REFERENCES

1. Kim HT. Vocal feminization for transgender women: current strategies and patient perspectives. Int J Gen Med 2020;13:43–52.
2. Xue SA, Cheng RW, Ng LM. Vocal tract dimensional development of adolescents: an acoustic reflection study. Int J Pediatr Otorhinolaryngol 2010;74(8):907–12.
3. Perry TL, Ohde RN, Ashmead DH. The acoustic bases for gender identification from children's voices. J Acoust Soc Am 2001;109(6):2988–98.
4. Nuyen B, Kandathil C, McDonald D, et al. The impact of living with transfeminine vocal gender dysphoria: Health utility outcomes assessment. Int J Transgender Health 2021. https://doi.org/10.1080/26895269.2021.1919277.
5. Seher S, Aslihan P, Firdevs A. Voice-related gender dysphoria: quality of life in hormone naïve trans male individuals. Anatolian J Psychiatry 2019;20:1.
6. Leung A, Tunkel A, Yurovsky D. Parents fine-tune their speech to children's vocabulary knowledge. Psychol Sci 2021;32(7):975–84.
7. Pelaez M, Virues-Ortega J, Gewirtz JL. Reinforcement of vocalizations through contingent vocal imitation. J Appl Behav Anal 2011;44(1):33–40.
8. WPATH. Standards of care for the health of transsexual, transgender, and gender nonconforming people [7th Version]. 2012. Available at: https://www.wpath.org/publications/soc.
9. American Speech-Language-Hearing Association (n.d. Voice and communication services for transgender and gender diverse populations. 2021. Available at: www.asha.org/Practice-Portal/Professional-Issues/Transgender-Gender-Diverse-Voice-and-Communication/.
10. Matthew M, Stoneham G. The voice book for trans and non-binary people: a practical guide to creating and sustaining authentic voice and communication. London: Jessica Kingsley Publishers; 2017.
11. Numerous authors. Trans affirming teacher referral list. Available at: https://docs.google.com/spreadsheets/d/1035WlnTLZ3dKT3BS6qt3itdR7So-bcRnvXwgTeCFajE/edit#gid=513350763.
12. American Speech-Language-Hearing Association. Standards and implementation procedures for the certificate of clinical competence in speech-language pathology. (Practice Portal). 2021. Available at: https://www.asha.org/certification/2020-slp-certification-standards/.

13. Tyack PL. A taxonomy for vocal learning. Philos Trans R Soc Lond B Biol Sci 2019; 375(1789):20180406.
14. Muhammad M, Wallerstein N, Sussman AL, et al. Reflections on researcher identity and power: the impact of positionality on community based participatory research (CBPR) processes and outcomes. Crit Sociol (Eugene) 2015;41(7–8): 1045–63.
15. Tschida K, Mooney R. The role of auditory feedback in vocal learning and maintenance. Curr Opin Neurobiol 2012;22(2):320–7.
16. Kinginger C. Enhancing language learning in study abroad. Annu Rev Appl Linguistics 2011;31:58–73.
17. Huang BH, Jun S-A. The effect of age on the acquisition of second language prosody. Language Speech 2011;54(3):387414.
18. Simpson AP. Dynamic consequences of differences in male and female vocal tract dimensions. J Acoust Soc Am 2001;109(5 Pt 1):2153–64.
19. Adler R, Hirsch S, Pickering J. Voice and communication therapy for the transgender/gender diverse client. San Diego, CA: Plural Publishing; 2019.
20. Davies S, Viktória G, Antoni C. Voice and communication change for gender nonconforming individuals: giving voice to the person inside. International J Transgenderism 2015;16(3):117–59.
21. Wolfe J, Garnier M, Smith J. Vocal tract resonances in speech, singing, and playing musical instruments. HFSP J 2009;3(1):6–23.
22. Kent RD, Vorperian HK. Static measurements of vowel formant frequencies and bandwidths: a review. J Commun Disord 2018;74:74–97.
23. Whalen DH, Chen WR, Tiede M, et al. Variability of articulator positions and formants across nine English vowels. J Phonetics 2018;68:1–14.
24. Neuhaus TJ. Gender perception dependent on fundamental frequency, source spectral tilt, and formant frequencies. Master's thesis. Bowling Green State University; 2020. Available at: http://rave.ohiolink.edu/etdc/view?acc_num= bgsu1586535654035042.
25. Garellek M, Samlan R, Gerratt BR, et al. Modeling the voice source in terms of spectral slopes. J Acoust Soc Am 2016;139(3):1404–10.
26. Sandy H. Combining voice, speech science and art approaches to resonant challenges in transgender voice and communication training. Perspect ASHA Spec Interest Groups 2017;2:74.
27. Uwe P, Simon G. Kinesthetic senses. Compr Physiol 2018;8(3):1157–83.

Feminization Laryngoplasty - A Comprehensive Approach to Reducing the Size of the Larynx and Pharynx

James Phillip Thomas, MD

KEYWORDS

- Feminization laryngoplasty • Femlar voice surgery • Transgender voice modification
- Pitch modification • Male-to-Female transition

KEY POINTS

- Auditory perception of femininity is related to pitch and resonance.
- Pitch is determined by the mass/length/tension of the vibrating edge.
- Resonance relates to supraglottic chamber area.

INTRODUCTION/HISTORY/DEFINITIONS/BACKGROUND
Feminization Laryngoplasty

Feminization laryngoplasty evolved from the aim to change a voice from a male quality to a female quality (**Figs. 1–13**). My suspicion is that a larynx and pharynx in a male has undergone enlargement during puberty and as there is no endocrine method for shrinking structures, a surgery that reduces the size of male structures to the size of female structures might alter the voice in an appropriate way. In theory, a smaller larynx and pharynx should raise both the fundamental frequency of the voice and the resonant frequency of the vocal tract. The initial attempts at this were undertaken in an attempt to address possible shortcomings in quality, longevity, as well as complications of existing procedures (cricothyroid approximation, vocal webbing, laser reduction).

On endoscopy in cis-gender individuals, male vocal cords seem longer and thicker than female, thus producing a lower comfortable speaking pitch and a lower lowest vocal pitch. There is usually a reduction of the upper vocal range and a change in the quality of the upper vocal range as thicker vocal cords must be stretched tighter to produce the same pitch as thinner, shorter cords.

Voicedoctor Private Practice, 909 Northwest 18th Avenue, Portland, OR 97209, USA
E-mail address: thomas@voicedoctor.net

Otolaryngol Clin N Am 55 (2022) 739–748
https://doi.org/10.1016/j.otc.2022.05.002
0030-6665/22/© 2022 Elsevier Inc. All rights reserved.

oto.theclinics.com

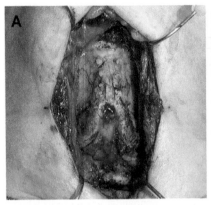
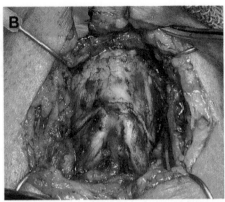

Fig. 1. (A) Exposed thyroid cartilage. (B) Marking the central thyroid cartilage and upper thyroid alae for removal of excess cartilage. (photos taken from point of view of the anesthetist. Rostral - bottom of photo. Caudal - top of photo.)

The relaxed laryngeal position drops lower in the neck in males, increasing the internal length of the pharyngeal chamber; a longer chamber selectively amplifies the lower notes via resonance. Even genetic females taking exogenous hormones, testosterone for libido or anabolic steroids for bodybuilding, often leads to the masculinization of the laryngeal structures.

In individuals identifying as female gender (whether genetically male, intersex, or cisfemale), self-practice or speech therapy may result in learning to produce a desirable speaking vocal pitch and resonance, masking changes induced by testosterone. These techniques use active compensatory muscle contraction of intrinsic and cervical muscles and require ongoing effort. Some individuals are successful in developing a habitual contraction, to the point of requiring little conscious effort to maintain laryngeal elevation for speaking with a female voice, while perhaps most others develop some fatigue from attempts at maintaining female pitch and resonance through tonic muscle contraction. Some individuals are unable to accomplish this task at all. Even when successful, many individuals remain fearful of letting their guard up for even a moment in a sensitive situation whereby an inadvertent masculine voice would be inappropriate.

This aids an individual in defining when to use speech therapy and when to consider surgery. For the individual who desires a feminine voice, who is interested in working

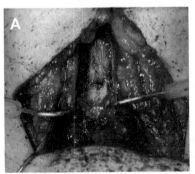
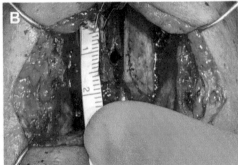

Fig. 2. Entering the airway. (A) Vocal ligaments are visible inferior to airway entry. (B) Vocal ligaments are at approximately 9-10 mm superior to the inferior margin of the thyroid cartilage.

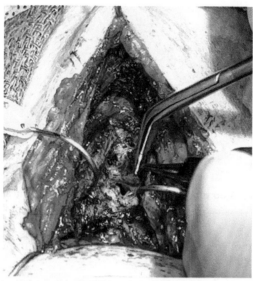

Fig. 3. False cords divided in the midline.

to achieve that goal, who isn't bothered by vocal fatigue or inadvertently slipping into a male voice, is highly risk intolerant then speech therapy is a reasonable approach, perhaps even the sole approach. But for the individual who never wants to sound male, speech therapy fails nearly 100% of the time. Without altering anatomy, there will be times when a male-quality voice will come out, even if only inadvertently. The individual will be constantly reminded throughout their life that they are transgender females.

Good candidates to consider anatomy altering procedures are:

1) The individual who never wants to sound male as only an approach that permanently alters anatomy has at least the possibility of achieving that goal.
2) The individual with poor vocal rapport
3) The individual who doesn't wish to spend time thinking and training.

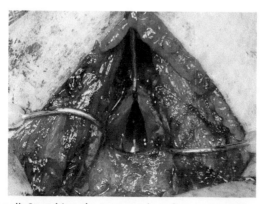

Fig. 4. Vocal cord pull. Stretching the true vocal cords to assess where to incise them for anterior excision.

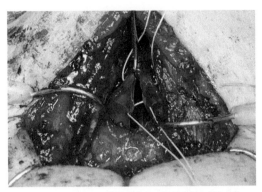

Fig. 5. Marking suture. A GoreTex suture has been placed marking the amount of true vocal cord to be preserved.

The potential cost of an anatomic-altering approach is that the individual needs to tolerate a number of risks:

1) The risk of surgical failure to achieve a female speaking pitch or a female vocal range
2) Associated costs of surgery,
3) Possible loss of speaking volume and
4) Even a poorer quality voice.

In the end though, in successful surgical approaches, the individual cannot sound male. Mentally, the postsurgical patient affirms the female gender during vocal intercourse. The transgender portion of life can be put behind them as a previous transitional phase.

Inspiration for the technique was drawn from the failures of cricothyroid approximation (falsetto/gay male vocal quality, loss of vocal range, return to the original pitch, loss of use of the cricothyroid muscle, locking into a single pitch) and an article by Somyos Kunachak.[1–3]

The guiding principle behind Feminization laryngoplasty is to convert as much of the larynx and pharynx to a more female morphology. The surgical approach is designed to:

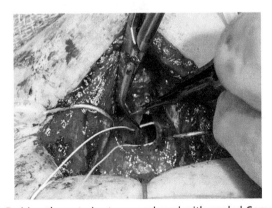

Fig. 6. True cord. Excising the anterior true vocal cord with angled Converse scissors.

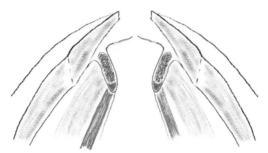

Fig. 7. Neocords post excision. Appearance of the true vocal cords after excision of the anterior portions.

1) Remove the anterior thyroid cartilage to collapse the area internal to the thyroid cartilage with the added benefit of removing the protruding profile of the Adam's Apple more extensively than the existing procedure of "Tracheal Shave."
2) Remove the anterior vocal cords to shorten the vocal cords, tension the vocal cords, and possibly thin the vocal cords by stretching them. The goal is to both raise the comfortable speaking pitch and remove the lower vocal range.
3) Shorten the false vocal cords narrowing the supraglottis, possibly altering resonance.
4) Remove the superior portion of the thyroid cartilage, shortening the vertical dimension of the larynx, and using thyrohyoid elevation suspend the larynx in a more typical female location, higher in the neck. The goal is internally shortening the pharyngeal chamber, altering resonance toward more feminine overtones.

DISCUSSION
Surgical Technique

A 5 to 8 cm incision is placed in or parallel to a skin crease directly in the midline. The incision is placed to easily reach from the cricothyroid membrane inferiorly to the hyoid bone superiorly. A longer incision allows easy reach and still looks cosmetically hidden if placed into a skin crease.

Strap muscles are separated in the midline exposing anatomy from the mid-hyoid bone to the upper cricothyroid membrane. Lateral dissection extends to the insertion of the thyrohyoid muscle onto the thyroid cartilage.

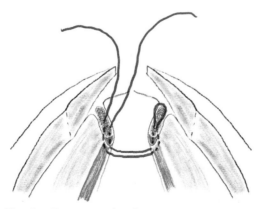

Fig. 8. First suture. First GoreTex suture placed to re-create the anterior commissure.

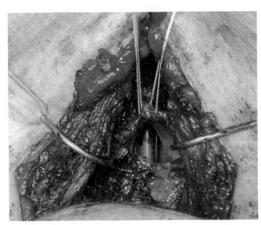

Fig. 9. Neo-glottis After placement of both GoreTex sutures, pulling on them recreates the anterior commissure.

The inferior border of the thyroid cartilage is superficially separated from the crico-thyroid membrane. There are frequently small arteries in the lateral portion of this area.

The midline is marked with a Bovie cautery and secondary marks are placed 2 to 4 mm lateral to the midline on each side. **Figure 1** I have removed as much as 8 mm of thyroid cartilage on each side of midline, but it can then be difficult to close a 16 mm gap in the midline as the internal lamina of the thyroid cartilage may abut the cricoid ring and prevent complete closure in the midline.

8 to 10 mm of the upper thyroid cartilage alae are excised. The remaining thyroid cartilage, when closed should more nearly resemble natal female thyroid cartilage in height and anterior apex angle.

The thyroid cartilage is divided vertically with an oscillating saw on either side of the midline with the saw kerf removing about one additional millimeter of cartilage.

The central, anterior thyroid cartilage is elevated away from the inner thyroid peri-chondrium and removed. The airway is not typically entered, though if it is, penetration usually occurs in the thinnest area, which is just superior to the anterior commissure. **Figure 2**.

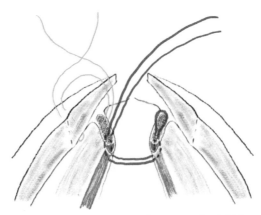

Fig. 10. TA suture. The green suture represents placement of a 4.0 Monocryl suture through the thyroarytenoid muscle and secured to the external thyroid laminae for direct tension on the anterior thyroarytenoid muscle.

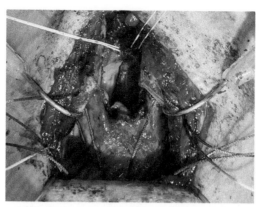

Fig. 11. TH elevation. Thyrohyoid sutures in place for elevation of the thyroid cartilage in the neck.

Removal of the vertical anterior thyroid cartilage segment will allow narrowing of the internal laryngeal aperture and very effectively removes the Adam's Apple contour (more completely than a "tracheal shave").

The airway is incised just superior to the anterior commissure, extending the midline incision superiorly through the anterior commissure of the false vocal cords. **Figure 3**

The anterior 5 mm of each false cord is excised, likely including the saccule. This reduces the diameter of the supraglottis after surgery. During surgery, this also provides an improved view of the true vocal cords and more space to manipulate needles within the larynx.

The anterior glottic ligament is pulled with a hook. **Figure 4** Assess how much of the anterior vocal cord needs to be removed to collapse the thyroid alae back into the midline while still maintaining tension on the vocal cords.

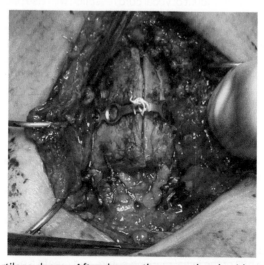

Fig. 12. Thyroid cartilage closure. After closure, the green thyrohyoid sutures have elevated the larynx in the neck. The microplate is secured with 4 mm screws in the lateral holes. The GoreTex sutures through the anterior commissure have been secured to the plate in the midline. The thyroid alae have been brought back to the midline.

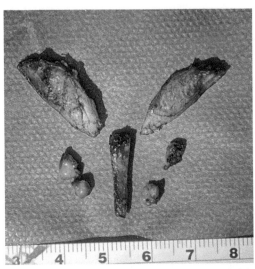

Fig. 13. Tissue removed. Thyroid cartilage, true vocal cord and false vocal cord tissue removed during the procedure. (Rostral - top of photo, Caudal - bottom of photo)

Stretch the true cords and use one-half of a double-ended CV-5 polytetrafluroethylene (Gore-Tex) suture to mark the perceived 50% location along the membranous vocal cords as measured from the anterior commissure. **Figure 5** I try to include the vocal ligament in this suture to maintain not only a symmetric anterior–posterior length to the neo-vocal cords but also to maintain the vibratory margins' vertical height symmetry. A usual goal is to remove about 40% of the anterior membranous vocal cord. With the removal of the anterior thyroid cartilage, the anterior–posterior dimension of the larynx will be smaller, so more membranous vocal cord must be removed to raise pitch than in a straight thyrotomy whereby only a small amount of vocal cord resection will raise pitch to some degree.

Tension of a cord by grasping the anterior vocal ligament and with angled scissors cut through the membranous cord. **Figure 6** The mucosal cuts are beveled from lateral to medial. **Figure 7** At the lateral aspect, the cut is at the edge of the inner lamina of the thyroid cartilage. Mucosa, vocal ligament, and the thyroarytenoid muscle are included in the removal. Bulky thyroarytenoid muscles may be stretched to remove a bit of additional muscle.

Using a Gore-Tex suture, enter the left thyroarytenoid muscle, passing through the vocal ligament (which feels slightly dense) and include about 1 mm of medial margin vocal cord epithelium. Attempt to exit at the upper vibratory lip of the membranous vocal cord. Pass into the opposite cord in a similar location beginning with the vocal cord epithelium and passing into the thyroarytenoid muscle. **Figure 8**

Return the needle back following an inferior path through the inferior vibratory lip of the membranous vocal cord, creating effectively a horizontal mattress suture into the vocal cords.

The removed marking suture is used as the opposing horizontal mattress suture starting in the right vocal cord, looping through the left, and returning to the right. When both of the horizontal mattress sutures are placed, tensioning them should nearly replicate the pull of the initial marking suture and create a new anterior commissure with shortened vocal cords. **Figure 9**

Additional pull on the thyroarytenoid muscle is helpful to keep it from retracting. A 4-0 Monocryl passed through the central aspect of the thyroarytenoid muscle and secured to the exterior of the thyroid cartilage sets the anterior muscle into place. **Figure 10** Loop the Monocryl through the muscle twice as muscle doesn't hold a suture as well as other tissue.

Muscles are elevated from the anterior inferior half of the hyoid bone with electrocautery for 10 mm on either side of the midline. 4 - 1 mm holes are drilled into the hyoid bone and 2 - 1 mm holes are drilled in the hyoid bone at four locations. Corresponding 1 mm holes are drilled into the upper cut edges of the thyroid cartilage, two holes on each side. Braided 0-Ethibond sutures are passed though the corresponding holes for later thyrohyoid elevation. **Figure 11**

To close the thyroid cartilage, 2, 1-mm holes are drilled in the new anterior edge of each thyroid cartilage, one inferior at the level of the subglottis, one superior at the level of the false vocal cords. 4-0 Monocryl sutures are passed through the cartilage, then through the cut ends of the false cords and out the opposite thyroid cartilage.

A second 4-0 Monocryl is passed through the inferior hole, through the subglottic cut edges of the inner perichondrium and out the opposite hole.

As the thyroid alae are held in approximation with forceps, the sutures are tied. The inferior suture is secondarily looped through the cricothyroid membrane snugging it up against the inferior thyroid cartilage. The upper suture is passed through the base of the epiglottis and snuggled up against the superior border of the thyroid cartilage. These sutures create additional seals preventing postoperative air leaks.

A micro-plate is curved to approximate the thyroid cartilage profile. The plate is secured at the location of the anterior commissure with the arms of the Gore-Tex sutures above and below. Self-tapping, 4 mm screws hold the plate and thyroid cartilage in place.

Gore-Tex is slippery enough to slide between even tightly approximated thyroid alae as it is cinched into place over the plate securing the new anterior commissure.

The Ethibond sutures pull the thyroid cartilage up close to the hyoid bone when tied, permanently elevating the larynx in the neck. Thyroid cartilage is positioned higher in the neck. Typically the thyroid cartilage is close to, but does not actually touch the hyoid bone. **Figure 12**

Strap muscles are reapproximated and can be slightly plicated, pulled superiorly, and reattached to the hyoid bone under some tension. Subcutaneous tissues are closed with 4-0 Monocryl. **Figure 13** shows removed tissue and cartilage.

OUTCOMES

Surgical outcomes have been detailed in two studies.[2,3] Audio files of postsurgical results are available for listening at https://www.voicedoctor.net/surgery/pitch-altering-surgeries/.[4]

CLINICS CARE POINTS

Location: Surgery can be performed at an outpatient surgical center.

Anesthesia: General endotracheal anesthesia, typically using a 6.0 endotracheal tube with a 2-h surgical time.

Antibiotics: For this clean-contaminated surgery a third-generation cephalosporin (cefotaxime - Claforan) or fluoroquinolone (levofloxacin - Levaquin) and clindamycin are administered.

Primary immediate postoperative risk: Because of the seriousness of airway swelling in the supraglottic region, postoperative antibiotics are given, the patient is examined endoscopically daily for 3 days. If swelling is resolving by the third day, supraglottic edema from infection is very unlikely.

Steroids: 10 mg dexamethasone at the time of surgery. Oral prednisone or methylprednisolone are given in selected cases if significant swelling develops postoperatively.

Recovery: Voice rest is requested for 2 weeks, although every patient coughs some, clears their throat, and may inadvertently speak, perhaps even in their sleep.

Avoid: no CPAP for the first 2 weeks. Air may leak from the closure creating subcutaneous emphysema, even from a cough. CPAP will make it much worse.

Voice: A few individuals have a great voice at 2 weeks. Most of the patients take 2 to 3 months to have enough swelling gone to assess whereby their voice is headed. It takes about 9 months before the voice is fully settled.

Revisions: revisions are possible, but most problems with the voice can be treated with laser approaches to the vocal cords.

Tracheal shave complication: Feminization laryngoplasty is an excellent approach to reattach and retighten vocal cords after vocal cord detachment.

Neck infections: If a neck becomes infected, it is likely the plate, screws and GoreTex sutures will need to be removed to clear the infection. These items are not needed for stability beyond about 30 days of healing.

Volume: almost all patients lose some or a moderate amount of volume.

SUMMARY

In Feminization Laryngoplasty, the thyroid cartilage and pharynx are shortened vertically. The true and false vocal cords are shortened by removing the anterior portions. Below the glottis, the cricoid cartilage remains unchanged. In successful cases, no further treatment is needed, typically including speech therapy. When pitch elevation and resonance change fail to match the female gender, there are often options to correct vocal cord oscillation further with additional laser procedures.

DISCLOSURE

The author has no commercial or financial conflicts of interest or any funding sources to disclose.

SUPPLEMENTARY DATA

Supplementary data related to this article can be found online at https://doi.org/10.1016/j.otc.2022.05.002.

REFERENCES

1. Kunachak S, Prakunhungsit S, Sujjalak K. Thyroid cartilage and vocal fold reduction: a new phonosurgical method for male-to-female transsexuals. Ann Otol Rhinol Laryngol 2000;109(11):1082–6.
2. Thomas JP, Macmillan C. Feminization laryngoplasty: assessment of surgical pitch elevation. Eur Arch Otorhinolaryngol 2013;270(10):2695–700.
3. Nuyen BA, Qian ZJ, Campbell RD, et al. Feminization Laryngoplasty: 17-Year Review on Long-Term Outcomes, Safety, and Technique. Otolaryngol Head Neck Surg 2021. https://doi.org/10.1177/01945998211036870. 1945998211036870.
4. Available at: https://www.voicedoctor.net/surgery/pitch-altering-surgeries/.

Voice and Speech Training for the Transgendered Patient

What the Otolaryngologist Should Know

Christella Antoni, MSc, BA Hons, HCPC, MRCSLT, MASLTIP[a,b,c,]*

KEYWORDS

- Speech/voice therapy • Speech therapy/pathology • Transgender
- Voice feminization • Glottoplasty

KEY POINTS

- Voice and speech are multifaceted phenomena.
- Transgender voice work is a subspecialist field of voice within speech pathology (SLP); the level and range of SLP experience with transgender voice are variable.
- Voice therapy treatment, for transgender and gender diverse people, is individualized according to each patient's goals.
- Voice therapy before and after voice feminization surgery can minimize dysphonia postsurgery.
- Indirect aspects of SLP intervention, such as psychosocial support to adjust to modified voice, can maximize outcomes for clients.

INTRODUCTION/HISTORY/DEFINITIONS/BACKGROUND

Voice therapy (VT) for transgender and gender diverse individuals is a specialized but growing field of speech and language therapy/pathology (SLT/P). The bulk of SLP intervention has typically been with the transfemale population (individuals assigned male at birth who identify as female), rather than with transmasculine clients (individuals assigned female at birth who identify as male). There are increasing indications that transmasculine individuals may benefit from SLP interventions,[1] including those who experience a slow rate of voice change or dysphonia following administration of hormones. However, the voice-lowering effects of testosterone achieve satisfactory

The author has no other funding, financial relationships, or conflicts of interest to disclose.
[a] University College London (UCL); [b] Chinese University of Hong Kong (CUHK); [c] Voice & Speech Services, 16 Middle Road, Harrow, Middlesex HA2 0HL, UK
* Corresponding author. Voice & Speech Services, 16 Middle Road, Harrow HA2 0HL, Middlesex, UK.
E-mail address: voice@christellaantoni.co.uk

voice outcomes for a high volume of transmen, and voice services are sought less frequently. In addition, SLP interventions with the transmasculine populations tend to be shorter, and far fewer transmen seek voice surgeries. For these reasons, this article more specifically discusses SLP interventions with transfemales, including those who seek voice feminization surgeries.

Voice and communication are complex physical phenomena influenced by a range of physical, behavioral, social, and emotional factors. However, the most researched aspect of transgender voice feminization is fundamental frequency (f0), the perceptual correlate of which is pitch.

DISCUSSION

Reliance on pitch measurement in transgender voice work occurs not least because f0 is measurable, unlike other voice aspects noted to be significant gender markers, such as resonance. The latter relies more on proprioception with traditional teaching relying more on artistic and perceptual experience.

f0 can be a defining aspect of female voice, but it is not the only aspect of successful female voice presentation. Intonation and aspects of articulation have also been identified as useful areas to target in VT.[2,3] Intonation and voice qualities and their close links with emotional expression can also significantly enhance female voice.

Although average speaking fundamental frequency (SFF) for women has been reported to be around 225 Hz,[4] this does not reflect the broad range of SFF found in cis-gendered women. Age contributes to pitch, with vocal pitch lowering noted in older women.[5] Higher SFF is found more commonly in younger women between 20 and 29 years of age.[6] Women in their 30s, 40s, and 50s are more often reported to have an SFF less than 200 Hz.[7] This allows for a variety of possibilities regarding pitch and transgender voice.

The critical f0 threshold for female voice identification has been identified as 155 to 160 Hz.[8,9] For individuals seeking a female-perceived voice outcome, targeting an average SFF of at least 155 Hz is therefore indicated. However, pitch and resonance are greatly influenced by each other. Raising the pitch uses thinner vocal folds, which in turn reduces chest resonance. By using more "forward focused" resonance (an increase in anterior oral and facial vibrations), higher pitch is more easily achieved and sustained. SLPs typically begin voice feminization development with resonance work, beginning with the nasal sound /m/, which clients can easily feel (by placing fingers on the side of their nose) and which can be combined with raised pitch as for making the sound of agreement /uhum/ or /mm/.

It is important to note that voice work is fear-inducing for most clients. Not only is there a sense that the task may seem insurmountable from a voice production perspective, but also it generally makes individuals feel self-conscious and uncomfortable. Part of the clinicians' skill lies in understanding the impact of vocal tract manipulations; "…pitch is not necessarily the result of high frequency but may be caused by the acoustic characteristics imparted to the voice by the supraglottic tract."[10] Furthermore, clinicians' skill lies in how to break down tasks into simple steps before gradually extending ability using hierarchically graded exercises. In addition, the psychosocial support aspects of transgender VT are little known outside of the remit of voice specialist SLP.

AMOUNT AND TYPE OF VOICE THERAPY RECEIVED

In standard (nontrans) VT, a typical course of treatment is approximately 6 sessions. In transgender VT, individuals can often achieve a gender-neutral voice in roughly the same timeframe. A female-perceived voice may be achieved in a similar treatment period, especially in reading tasks. Typically, however, sustaining voice in all social contexts requires additional sessions. There are clients who achieve consistent female voice in less sessions (audio voice samples can be accessed on www.christellaantoni. co.uk).[11] However, quick voice change is less common than a slower pace of voice modification. Although development of further vocal stamina may be indicated, a more common issue is that clients feel self-conscious about using altered voice. Progressing through this unsure phase is necessary for most individuals before becoming comfortable with using modified voice.

Thousands of female voice outcomes with transwomen have demonstrated to this author that an optimal amount of voice sessions is approximately 12 sessions. The voice program needs to be comprehensive, with gaps between sessions approximately 2 weeks apart and not more than 4 weeks apart if possible. This allows for steady progress and consistent SLP support during treatment.

The amount and type of VT received can therefore be extremely significant. In many publicly funded health systems, VT sessions may be limited to between 4 and 6 sessions, and the gaps are often 4 weeks or more. For example, the SLT department of the United Kingdom's Tavistock and Portman's Gender Identity Clinic now offers "up to four one to one" sessions, spaced at monthly intervals.[11] (Waiting lists in national health services tend to be growing with some clients waiting up to 4 years for an initial assessment with a clinician.) A limited amount of treatment sessions, large gaps between sessions, together with varying levels of experience among treating clinicians, may lead to limited outcomes for clients.

Services constrained to offering a limited amount of treatment sessions impact clinicians' ability to develop advanced skills, as the skills are built on each other over time. Clinicians with more extensive voice expertise and specific training in transgender voice can typically gain clients' confidence more easily. This in turn may mean clients move more effectively through treatment, particularly through the bridging exercises from "practice voice" to "actual everyday voice."

It is in the latter stages of VT that longer and more complex exercises are possible, such as voice projection, telephone voice, and sustained conversation tasks. (Aspects such as feminizing cough, laugh, yawn, and sneezing may be worked on during later stages of treatment if indicated/required by the client.) More advanced exercises assist with facilitating secure and flexible voice ability over time. Many clients cite lack of ability to project their female voice or report being misidentified on the telephone. Reassuring clients that the ability very often increases as the later stage exercises are practiced helps to lessen anxieties (**Table 1**).

It is also important to note that dysphonia can be a presenting issue in at least one-quarter of trans clients presenting for voice modification work, a finding also reported by other clinicians.[12] However, SLP experience working with standard voice caseloads before beginning transgender voice work is becoming less prevalent. This can potentially limit optimal vocal functioning for trans clients. Conversely, clinicians who primarily have experience working with dysphonia but very little opportunity to work with trans voice may lack the cultural competence and range of voice exercises required to achieve voice modification. For example, a perseveration on breath, relaxation, and straw phonation work proves largely ineffective when aiming to modify pitch or intonation.

The issue of postgraduate training in SLP is an area of concern in certain services. As a trainer of SLPs in standard voice and transgender voice work since 2002, the author has noted more UK clinicians in the National Health Service self-fund or partial fund their training rather than be funded by their local health authority/department. In

Table 1 Staged voice therapy treatment program (Antoni method)		
Stage 1	**Initial Level Exercises**	**Monitoring and Possible Outcome**
	• Including resonance, pitch, intonation	• Baseline perceptual and pitch measures made (initial assessment)
	• Up to short sentence level (reading)	• End stage 1 voice recordings made
	• Short length conversation practice	• Gender-neutral voice may be achieved (more often in reading only)
Stage 2:	Intermediate level exercises	
	• Including prosody, vocal tone lightening, intonation variation articulation modifications	
	• Longer length reading tasks	• End stage 2 voice recordings made
	• Extending conversation practice	• Gender neutral: feminine voice may be achieved in reading and speaking
Stage 3:	Advanced level exercises, including	
	• Vocal tone brightening (supraglottic adjustments)	
	• Voice projection	
	• Intensity flexibility	
	• Increasing vocal stamina (both reading and speaking voice)	End of stage 3 voice recordings made
	• Telephone voice	Female voice presentation may be achieved[a]

[a] Note: Some clients may achieve their voice goals in less sessions/stages. Others may require additional sessions. Options for additional sessions and/or voice surgery are reviewed during the therapy process.

general, a stark paucity of clinicians with experience of managing before and after voice feminization surgeries exists.

PSYCHOSOCIAL CONSIDERATIONS

Counseling forms a significant part of a voice specialist SLP's work, from working with clients experiencing voice loss, psychogenic voice cases, and especially when working with transgender voice. "Trans women who reported greater difficulties and voice-related effects in their lives had more symptoms of anxiety and depression."[13]

Adjustment to using modified voice is also a subject that receives little attention. Most clients do not go from one voice to another without overcoming barriers. Self-doubt can consistently threaten the process. Habituation of the modified voice requires the client to walk a dual path: working through presenting barriers while also continuing to develop vocal ability. A dual track approach taken by clinicians will also limit potential derailing of the voice change process: managing clients' emotional vocal challenges while continuing along the VT program.

Increasing clients' awareness of the stages of voice modification assists in managing expectations. Without this awareness, clients and clinicians can often feel they are making inadequate progress or that further voice modification is not possible.

Additional possible psychosocial aspects that may affect progress of voice modification are as follows:

- Limited social experience in the client's preferred gender. Transfeminine clients who wish to make a female social transition but lack lived experience tend to benefit from additional VT sessions.
- Lower levels of perceptual awareness. Clinicians who are diligent with obtaining voice recordings and pitch measures at the start and at various stages during treatment can significantly increase the client's perceptual awareness. In many cases, a successful VT process also involves desensitizing clients to the sound of their voice, at least to some degree. Although most people experience sensitivity listening to their voice, for the trans individual, it can be a particular source of vocal dysphoria.
- Mental health challenges
- Anxieties manifesting as vocal dysphoria (conversion symptoms). A case example follows.

A client previously happy with her postglottoplasty voice progress became severely vocally dysphoric after a few months, citing a pitch decrease. Other issues in the client's life were explored by the therapist during the session. The client became emotional describing her imminent trip overseas to see her family, none of whom had seen her in since her transition. The client was able to make a connection between the emotional pressure of this impending event and her growing dissatisfaction with her postsurgical voice.

- General low confidence levels

Time, effort, and often expense are inherent in the process of successful voice modification. For these reasons, and the difficulty clients sometimes experience accessing, committing to, or benefiting from VT, clients may seek surgical interventions to assist voice change. Even in cases where voice change has been significant with VT alone, the client's vocal anxiety may remain high. Their hope is that these anxieties will be alleviated with voice surgery.

VOICE FEMINIZATION SURGERIES

The increased availability of glottoplasty has assisted many transwomen. Pitch elevation following surgery has been described by a range of investigators.[14–16] Clients have reported increased quality of life using measures such as VHI-10 and the Trans Woman Voice Questionnaire.[15,17]

Reduced vocal dysphoria and increased vocal confidence postsurgery are common. However, for some individuals, vocal anxiety can remain high following surgery. This may be due to factors such as clients pinning all vocal hopes into the surgery and postsurgery dysphonia. A pitch increase alone may not be enough for the client to perceive their voice as female. A study by Mora and colleagues found "No correlation exists between increase in $f0$ and improvement of SPFV (self-perceived female voice) or increase of $f0$ and improvement of QoL rv (quality of life related to voice) either after CTA or GL and increases in $F0$." Only clients who had not received any previous VT were included in this study, which could potentially show the pure effects of surgery alone. However, the lack of SLP input may have been a contributory factor to the reported lack of SPVF and QoL rv outcomes related to $f0$.

In the author's 21 years' experience, clients who undergo a course of VT presurgery and postsurgery tend to fare better postsurgically. A presurgery course of treatment, at least up to intermediate exercise level, benefits the client in a range of ways described above. In addition, as glottoplasty primarily assists with raising average pitch and may result in a reduction of dynamic range, an initial course of therapy

---

Box 1
Recommended voice therapy interventions before and after voice feminization surgery

Presurgery:
• Client to complete at least short course of voice therapy
• Presurgery assessment with SLT, including voice recordings: perceptual & f0; postsurgery voice care advice given
• Postsurgery voice rehabilitation session or sessions booked

Postsurgery Stage 1:
• Voice rehabilitation sessions booked starting 10 to 14 days postsurgery (4 × 25-minute sessions recommended)
• Postsurgery voice recordings: perceptual & f0;
• Client subjective evaluation of voice: discussed with SLP
• Counseling support if indicated
• Liaison with voice surgeon

Postsurgery stage 2 (optional, according to clients' goals):
• Continued voice rehabilitation if indicated
• Intermediate: advanced voice therapy exercises (eg, to assist with aspects such as developing vocal stamina and voice projection)
• Client subjective evaluation of voice
• Voice recordings–perceptual and f0
• Liaison with voice surgeon

---

will also provide an opportunity to develop female voice characteristics, such as increased use of intonation and intonation range.[18,19] These and additional aspects, when combined with raised pitch, potentially produce a more natural sounding, flexible female voice.

Following having performed a glottoplasty, the author recommends a course of VT specifically for voice rehabilitation beginning 10 to 14 days postsurgery. Ideally, these voice rehabilitation sessions will be shorter in length than standard length sessions (approximately 25 minutes), as vocal fatigue and hoarseness postsurgery are present to varying degrees for up to 6 weeks in many cases. Following the voice rehabilitation sessions, clients can continue with additional sessions to assist with developing aspects such as increased ability to project voice safely (**Box 1**).

In addition, postsurgery VT can assist the client with psychological adjustment to the postsurgical voice. The client may relate feelings of "unsureness" about the postsurgical voice or finding it "hard to get used to." *The value of VT to help clients release laryngeal tension cannot be underestimated.* Vocally self-conscious individuals are more likely to constrict the voice to varying degrees in the larynx: "place" their voice in the throat. This exacerbates roughness in the voice and prevents safe voice projection. Increased dysphonia and loss of vocal power have been described as possible voice "tradeoffs" for pitch increases gained via glottoplasty.[20] They are often easily remediated with appropriate clinical guidance.

FUTURE DIRECTIONS

With the advancing availability of voice feminization surgeries, it is likely that more transfeminine clients will seek surgical interventions. Building and developing links between surgeons and clinicians can only help to maximize potential results for clients. Recent studies evaluating surgical techniques and outcomes have helped to inform our practice.[21,22] Further investigations will continue to help us refine our clinical and surgical interventions.

Although empirical evidence may be high in some services, systematic reviews on the effectiveness of voice training for transwomen are limited. An increase in evaluation of different VT programs could inform clinical practice significantly. The few studies at research hierarchy level 2 appear to demonstrate the effectiveness of voice training.[23,24] The research issue is further compounded by the individualized approach taken by clinicians as indicated by their respective clients' goals. Oates reminds us that transwomen are not a homogenous population and that "[t]his heterogeneity makes scientific control difficult and can limit the feasibility and value of randomised control trials."[25,26]

Although the number of voice therapists who specialize in transgender and gender diverse voice is on the increase, advanced specialists are still limited. Even more limited are the voice specialists with experience of working with prevoice and postvoice feminization surgery. Expert level practitioners can help to support less-experienced voice therapists.

SUMMARY

Transgender voice work can be equally challenging and rewarding. All voice journeys are unique and require a nuanced level of support. As a relatively new field, practice will continue to be informed by future clinical endeavors and joint working. Assisting clients who seek gender identity and voice alignment ultimately enhances their social comfort and functioning.

CLINICS CARE POINTS

- Speech pathologists work with clients' own self-defined goals. This may include working with clients to help them achieve a voice that is perceived as female, male, or gender neutral.
- Although pitch can be an important gender marker, voices can be perceived as female from 155 to 160 Hz.
- Transfemales seeking a female-perceived voice are recommended to complete a comprehensive staged treatment program with a suitably skilled clinician.
- Voice therapy involves practicing exercises with clients coupled with therapeutic counseling support.
- A higher pitch/satisfaction voice may not necessarily ensue following voice feminization surgery if clients adopt a suboptimal voicing pattern.
- Voice surgery outcomes may be maximized with before and after voice therapy interventions.

REFERENCES

1. Davies S, Papp V, Antoni C. Voice and communication change for gender nonconforming individuals: Giving Voice to the person inside. Int J Transgenderism 2015;16:117–59.
2. Oates JM, Dacakis G. Transgender voice & communication: research evidence underpinning voice interventions for male-to-female transsexual women. Perspect Voice Voice Disord 2015;25(2):48.
3. Andrews ML. Manuel of voice treatment, paediatrics through geriatrics. San Diego (CA): Singular Publishing; 1999.
4. Greene M, Mathieson L. The voice & its disorders. 6th edition. London, U.K: Whurr Publishers; 2001.

5. Antoni C, Sandhu G. Gender dysphoria and the larynx. In: Costello D, Sandhu G, editors. Practical laryngology. Boca Raton (FL): Taylor Francis; 2016.
6. Stoiceff M. Speaking fundamental frequency characteristics on non-smoking female adults. J Speech Hear Res 1981;24:437–41.
7. Colton R, Casper JK, Leonard R. Understanding voice problems. A physiological perspective for diagnosis and treatment. 3rd edition. Baltimore (MD): Lippincott Williams and Wilkins; 2006.
8. Spencer L. Speech characteristics of male-to-female transsexuals: a perceptual and acoustic study. Folia Phoniatr 1988;40:31–42.
9. Wolfe VL, Ratusnik DL, Smith FH, et al. Intonation and fundamental frequency in male-to-female transsexuals. J Speech Hear Disord 1990;55:43–50.
10. Greene M, Mathieson L. The voice and its disorders. 6th edition. London (UK): Whurr Publishers; 2001.
11. Available at: http://www.christellaantoni.co.uk.
12. Available at: http://gic.nhs.uk.
13. Hancock AB, Garabedian LM. Transgender voice & communication treatment: a retrospective chart review of 25 cases. Int J Lang Commun Disord 2013;45(5): 313–24.
14. Novais Valente Junior C, Mesquita de Medeiros A. Voice and gender incongruence: relationship between vocal self-perception and mental health of trans women. J Voice 2020.
15. Brown SK, Chang J, Hu S, et al. Addition of Wendler glottoplasty to voice therapy improves trans female voice outcomes. Laryngoscope 2021;131(7):1588–93.
16. Ramacle M, Matar N, Morsomme D, et al. Glottoplasty for male-to-female transsexualism: voice results. J Voice 2011;25(1):120–3.
17. Yilmaz T, Ozer F, Aydinli FE. Laser reduction glottoplasty for voice feminisation: experience on 28 patients. Ann Otol Rhinol Laryngol 2021;130(9):1057–63.
18. Mora E, Cobeta I, Becerra A, et al. Comparison of cricothyroid approximation and glottoplasty for surgical voice feminisation in male-to-female transsexuals. Laryngoscope 2018;128:2101–9.
19. Gelfer & Schofield 2013.
20. Hancock A, Colton L, Douglas F. Intonation and gender perception: applications for transgender speakers. J Voice 2014;28:203–9.
21. Titze IR, Palaparthi A, Mau T. Vocal tradeoffs in anterior glottoplasty for voice feminisation. Laryngoscope 2020;00:1–7.
22. Schwartz K, Fantanari AMV, Scheider MA, et al. Laryngeal surgical in transgender women: a systematic review and meta analysis. Laryngoscope 2017;127(11): 2596–603.
23. Song TE, Jiang N. Transgender phonosurgery: a systematic review and meta-analysis. Otolaryngol Head Neck Surg 2017;156:803–8.
24. Gelfer MP, Tice RM. Perceptual and acoustic outcomes of voice therapy for male-to-female transsexuals perceived as female versus those perceived as male. J Voice 2013;27:335–47.
25. Gelfer MP, Van Dong BR. A Preliminary Study on the use of vocal function exercises to improve voice in male-to-female transgender clients. J Voice 2013;27: 321–34.
26. Oates J. M. In Adler, H & Pickering J (editors). Evidence-based practice in voice training for trans women. Voice and communication therapy for the transgender/gender diverse client. a comprehensive clinical guide, (3rd edition). (pp.87-103). San Diego, CA, Plural Publishing.

Masculinization Laryngoplasty

C. Michael Haben, MD, MSc

KEYWORDS

• Voice • Speech • Male • Masculine • Transgender • Testosterone

KEY POINTS

• Up to 20% of transgendered males on testosterone therapy fail to achieve a voice that is sufficiently masculine even after sufficient speech therapy.
• Masculinization laryngoplasty is an effective procedure to reduce pitch.
• Pitch reduction laryngeal framework surgery is also useful in non-transgendered patients with high-pitched voice disorders.

CLINICAL RELEVANCE

There exist several clinical situations where the speaking fundamental frequency of an individual is higher than expected or desired. These high-pitched voice disorders may be caused by intrinsic vocal fold issues such as scarring and sulci or developmental issues including the infantile larynx and mutational falsetto (puberphonia). Over the last couple of decades, there has been a shift in the percentage of patients who present with a voice that is too high to align with their perceived, desired, or affirmed identity despite having a voice and speaking frequency that would otherwise be appropriate for their birth gender. Female-to-male transgendered persons make up the bulk of this population; however, certain cisgendered men as well as persons identifying as nonbinary, inter-gendered, "butch lesbian" women, and "gay" men are presenting with dysphoria secondary to voice characteristics that are not congruent with their identity perception, prompting them to seek out a more masculine voice.

INTRODUCTION

Voice has been identified as one of the most overt dimorphic traits playing a leading role in both perceived and attributed gender identity. In the transgendered male population, a masculine voice has been rated as one of the traits patients who were least satisfied with before initiation of masculinizing-gender-affirming hormone therapy (M-

Director, Center for the Care of the Professional Voice, 980 Westfall Road, Rochester, NY 14618, USA
E-mail address: Michael.Haben.MD@professionalvoice.org

Otolaryngol Clin N Am 55 (2022) 757–765
https://doi.org/10.1016/j.otc.2022.04.011
0030-6665/22/© 2022 Elsevier Inc. All rights reserved.

oto.theclinics.com

GAHT) and ranked as the "most important" anticipated change once therapy had begun.[1] The development of a masculine voice is a fundamental part of transition in transgendered men as well as an essential part of gender identity in cisgendered men.[2] Numerous studies have established that the speaking fundamental frequency (F_0) of both cisgendered and transgendered speakers is probably the greatest, albeit far from the lone, acoustic parameter in perceived and attributed gender identity.[3–5] Pitch reduction may be accomplished by several therapies. These include speech and voice training, hormonal treatments, and surgical procedures. Detailed information regarding transgender voice retraining/speech therapy and GAHT may be found in other articles of this issue.

First-line therapy for high-pitched voice disorders in cisgendered patients is generally speech therapy. In transgendered men, M-GAHT frequently in a combination of voice retraining with laryngeal repositioning[6] is considered the first-line standard of care. The mainstay of M-GAHT is testosterone. The impact of M-GAHT, testosterone specifically, on the voice, has been well-documented.[7] After initiation of M-GAHT, voice deepening is expected within 3 to 12 months, and a maximum benefit is typically realized by 1 to 2 years.[8] It has been reported that although some testosterone-naïve transgendered men experience voice lowering within the first 3 months of testosterone therapy initiation, the majority will experience changes to the voice between 6 and 9 months.[9] Although most of the transgendered men treated with testosterone (with or without speech training) can expect a lowering of their pitch, a percentage of patients report that the degree of pitch reduction is insufficient to result in a voice that is perceived as belonging to a male.[10] Insufficient pitch reduction, either subjectively or objectively, has been reported in approximately 20% of transgendered men receiving appropriate M-GAHT for an adequate duration of time.[11] This suboptimal response seems to be associated with diminished androgen sensitivity.[12] The degree to which voice changes occur on testosterone therapy may also depend on the age at which M-GAHT is initiated. In transgendered men who do not achieve cisgender male frequencies (defied as $F_0 \leq 131$ Hz) after 1 to 2 years of adequate M-GAHT or have voices not perceived as being sufficiently masculine despite a reasonable trial of voice retraining, pitch reduction laryngeal framework surgery may be considered to lower F_0.

Laryngeal framework surgery has been performed for decades. The seminal work by Isshiki in 1974[13] described and codified the four basic types of thyroplasty procedures: type I, "lateral compression", used for correction of glottic insufficiency, commonly augmentation or medialization laryngoplasty, such as is performed for unilateral vocal fold paralysis; type II, "lateral expansion", used for correction of vocal fold hyperadduction, commonly posterior cordectomy or lateralization laryngoplasty, such as is performed for bilateral vocal fold immobility; type III, "relaxation of vocal cord", used for pitch reduction, such as is performed for high-pitched voice disorders; and type IV, "stretching of vocal cord", used for pitch elevation, commonly glottoplasty and cricothyroid approximation, such as is performed for androphonia. Detailed information on feminization laryngoplasty may be found elsewhere in this issue. In 2001, the European Laryngological Society expanded Isshiki's classification of "thyroplasty" to incorporate procedures not solely limited to the thyroid cartilage under the new heading of laryngeal framework surgery to include different procedures having the same intent to approximate (type 1), expand (type 2), relax (type 3), and tense (type 4) the vocal fold(s) for varying voice outcomes.[14]

Outcome data sets for Isshiki thyroplasty type III (IT3) for pitch lowering specifically in transgendered men are just beginning to be published. In one study,[15] eight transgendered men undergoing IT3 had their F_0 drop significantly from the preoperative mean of 154.60 ± 12.29 Hz to the postoperative mean of 105.37 ± 10.52 Hz ($t = 9.821, P < .001$).

Anecdotally, an average of approximately 50 Hz of pitch reduction may be achieved in most patients undergoing IT3 in the author's unpublished experience with 44 female-to-male transgendered patients. A predecessor of the Isshiki type III thyroplasty has been reported as early as 1973[16] in the treatment of high-pitched voice disorders related to sulcus vocalis where only an anterior commissure + thyroid cartilage attachment window is developed and posteriorly displaced. Other applications of this technique have been described for refractory and recalcitrant high-pitched voice disorders in cisgendered men with mutational falsetto. Pitch reduction for high-pitched voice disorders related to sulcus vocalis has been reported in the range of 60 Hz[17] and up to 140 Hz[18] for mutational voice disorders. The Isshiki type III thyroplasty seems capable of lowering fundamental frequency of speech without adversely affecting the vibratory mode of the vocal folds in terms of acoustic parameters of jitter and shimmer quotients, vocal intensity, or vocal fold movement.[19]

EVALUATION

In the care of the transgendered population, gender-affirming surgery of the head and neck is considered an irreversible intervention. This includes pitch-lowering laryngeal framework surgery.

As an international multidisciplinary organization setting the standards for care of transgendered individuals, The World Professional Association of Transgender Health in its most recent Standards of Care publication (SOC 7, published in 2012) strongly recommended that patients considering genital ("bottom") surgery have not only a persistent, well-documented history of gender dysphoria, but also completed 12 continuous months of hormonal therapy. There are no explicit recommendations in SOC 7 for behavioral health documentation or duration of hormonal therapy before pitch reduction laryngoplasty; however, most providers would consider "living as the affirmed gender" and on appropriate M-GAHT for a minimum of 1 year with an adequate trial of voice retraining before considering a patient a reasonable candidate for irreversible surgery. Transgendered patients frequently undergo several gender-affirming surgical procedures as part of their transition. In transgendered men, these may include genitoplasty, mastectomies, body sculpting/implants, facial masculinization, and masculinization voice surgery. It is not uncommon for transgendered patients to get as many procedures done in the shortest time span to speed up their transition and address their gender dysphoria. The timing of masculinization laryngoplasty should be taken into consideration relative to other procedures under general endotracheal intubation. Some surgeons, including the author, recommend against general endotracheal intubation for elective procedures for at least 3 months following masculinization laryngoplasty to prevent accidental displacement of the cartilage during the postoperative period based on anecdotal experience from laryngeal fractures.

Preoperative evaluation by a qualified speech–language pathologist is beneficial both in terms of high-quality baseline acoustic parameters and in helping patients understand the important acoustic parameters that are not expected to change after pitch-lowering masculinization laryngeal framework surgery. These voice characteristics, specifically the rate of speech and sound pressure levels, have been shown to have an impact on voice masculinity and gender attribution.[20] Preprocedure initiation of speech therapy permits patients to focus on surgically non-alterable voice parameters in addition to addressing pitch.

Routine preoperative laboratories and/or imaging are not routinely recommended in most patients without specific risk factors; however, in those where blood tests have been obtained, the clinician should be aware of the impact that M-GAHT testosterone

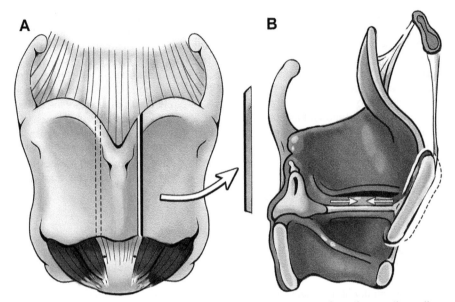

Fig. 1. Type III thyroplasty involves removal of a 1 to 2 mm strip of cartilage unilaterally or bilaterally (*curved arrow*) at approximately 3 mm lateral to the midline (*A*) allowing tension of the ipsilateral or bilateral vocal fold(s) (*double arrows*) to be reduced (*B*). Figure by Chynna DeSimone

therapy has on the presence of erythrocytosis. In addition, increases in ALT and AST are not uncommon, especially in the first year after initiation of M-GAHT. The author recommends smoking and nicotine cessation (including e-cigarettes, cannabis, vaping, pipes, and chewed tobacco) for a minimum of 3 months preoperatively and 6 months to permanently postoperatively. In patients who smoke and are known to have erythrocytosis, smoking cessation is recommended for a minimum of 6 months preoperatively to be deemed a reasonable candidate. Additional information on GAHT is found elsewhere in this issue.

SURGICAL TECHNIQUES

Pitch-lowering laryngoplasty is primarily based on the concept of reducing tension on the vocal folds. The various techniques used, including the three described here, are variations of an Isshiki type III thyroplasty and fall under the nomenclature of "relaxation" laryngoplasty using the European Laryngological Society's proposal. Each of these procedures has been described as being amenable to either local anesthesia with or without sedation or general anesthesia. The advantages of local sedation include the ability to perform intraoperative monitoring of pitch reduction and vocal quality as well as intraoperative transnasal laryngoscopy. In each of these techniques, the approach is essentially identical. The patient is in the supine position with the head extended. Preoperative prophylactic antibiotics and steroids (Decadron 10 mg IVP) are administered. A midline, horizontal cervical incision is made in a skin crease overlying the thyroid cartilage. The strap muscles are divided into the midline raphé and retracted laterally. The thyroid cartilage is exposed from the superior to the inferior border. The outer perichondrium is divided and preserved.

In a description for clinical application by Isshiki,[21] the type III thyroplasty involves removal of a 1 to 2 mm strip of cartilage unilaterally at approximately 3 mm lateral to the midline (**Fig. 1**A) allowing tension of the ipsilateral vocal fold to be reduced (**Fig. 1**B). Originally, if insufficient reduction of tension is achieved, the procedure may be expanded on the ipsilateral side by increasing the width of the strip removed or performed concurrently on the contralateral side. Isshiki stated that pitch-lowering effect was much greater when performed on both sides. Currently, unilateral utilization of an IT3 for masculinization in transgendered patients is not commonly performed.

Clinical Note: for each of these surgical approaches, preservation of the inner thyroid perichondrium is of the utmost importance.

In the modified Isshiki type III (medial approach, sometimes referred to as type IIIB) technique, a window is prepared over the midline keeping the anterior commissure centered.[22] Once the anterior commissure–thyroid cartilage complex is appropriately developed (**Fig. 2**A), it may be retrodisplaced with a reduction of tension on the vocal folds (**Fig. 2**B). Potential advantages of this approach include the integrity of the remaining thyroid cartilage, which is otherwise separated into three pieces in a bilateral Isshiki type III thyroplasty. In addition to greater stability, the height of the thyroid notch is maintained. A loss of prominence of the "Adam's Apple" could be a source of dysphoria in both cisgendered and transgendered men.

The approach preferred by the author is a different modification of the Isshiki type III thyroplasty where instead of separating the thyroid cartilage into three pieces with the removal of two lateral strips: a "second-class lever" is developed with the fulcrum centered at the inferior thyroid cartilage and the median cricothyroid ligament. The thyrotomies are performed using a 2-mm oscillating bone saw 3 mm lateral to the midline on each side (**Fig. 3**A). No strip of cartilage is removed. The medial portion is subluxed under the lateral portions once the inner perichondrium of the lateral portions has been elevated for 2 mm (**Fig. 3**B). The justification for this approach is related to the anatomy

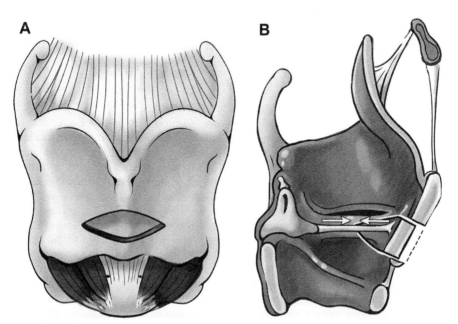

Fig. 2. Once the anterior commissure–thyroid cartilage complex is appropriately developed (*A*) it may be retrodisplaced with a reduction of tension on the vocal folds (*B*). Figure by Chynna DeSimone

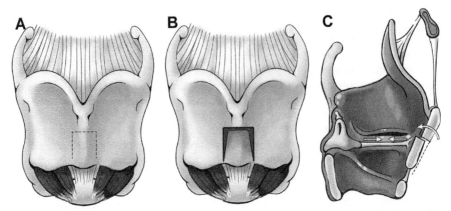

Fig. 3. The thyrotomies are performed using a 2-mm oscillating bone saw 3 mm lateral to the midline on each side. (*A*) No strip of cartilage is removed. The medial portion is subluxed under the lateral portions once the inner perichondrium of the lateral portions has been elevated for 2 mms. (*B*) The anterior commissure–thyroid cartilage complex from the rest of the thyroid structure (*C*). Figure by Chynna DeSimone

of the conus elasticus. In the author's experience, developing a second-class lever allows a greater control over tension on the vocal ligament and permits a wider range of anterior commissure retrodisplacement without complete separation of the anterior commissure–thyroid cartilage complex from the rest of the thyroid structure (**Fig. 3C**). The degree of applied force (subluxation) may be measured by intraoperative subjective or objective voice analysis as well as transnasal laryngoscopy in a non-intubated patient. Once an optimal position has been achieved, the medial portion may be secured using horizontal mattress sutures incorporating the outer perichondrium when possible. This approach also prevents the loss of lateral projection and prominence of the thyroid notch associated with the classic bilateral IT3.

CASE REPORT

A 36-year-old transgendered man presents with inappropriately high voice resulting in dysphoria, despite an adequate trial of testosterone cypionate 50 mg subcutaneous injection each week for almost 2 years. On this dose of M-GAHT, the patient achieved amenorrhea within 3 months as well as the development of oily skin, acne, and some androgenic hair loss within the first year. Facial and body hair virilization was also noted within the first 12 months as was some deepening of the voice, however, these changes plateaued despite several changes to the testosterone dosing and administration. A 9-month trial of voice therapy with an experienced speech–language pathologist was ineffective to improve his dysphoria. The patient presented to the author with a preoperative speaking fundamental frequency of 165 Hz. Documented pre-GAHT F_0 was reportedly 185 Hz. The patient underwent an uncomplicated modification of the Isshiki type III thyroplasty using the "second-class lever" technique described above under general anesthesia with bilateral infraglottic augmentation vocal fold injections using a permanent biocompatible material increasing vocal fold density. Preoperative and postoperative day 1 laryngeal images are shown in **Fig. 4**, respectively. Analysis of a patient-provided 3-month postoperative voice recording of the Rainbow Passage demonstrated an F_0 of 110 Hz. The patient reports resolution

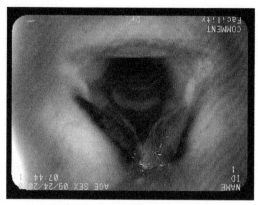

Fig. 4. Preoperative and postoperative day 1 laryngeal images.

of his dysphoria and "zero" episodes of being misgendered over the telephone. The 55-Hz pitch reduction was roughly the average expected.

POSTOPERATIVE CARE

The author recommends 14 days of postoperative voice rest. The justification for this recommendation is related to the degree of subepithelial ecchymosis frequently noted in postoperative laryngoscopy, which is treated like that of severe bilateral vocal fold hemorrhage.[23]

An ice pack to the anterior neck for the first week helps with postoperative discomfort and edema. Narcotic pain control is generally not necessary.

In addition to steroids and antibiotics, patients are placed on showering restrictions for 7 days (until the running subcuticular skin suture is removed) and instructed to avoid lifting anything greater than 5 pounds for 30 days. Patients are instructed to abstain from contact sports and elective procedures with general endotracheal intubation for 3 months. Patients are also advised to disclose to future surgical and anesthesia teams that they have had a masculinization laryngoplasty in the past.

OUTCOMES

In general, pitch reduction in experienced hands may be consistently achieved, with many clients realizing up to 50 to 60 Hz lowering, and an F_0 within the range of cisgendered men. Postprocedure outcome data in transgendered men are just beginning to be reported. One consideration for current data sets is the use of visual analog scales in this population who frequently have no baseline laryngeal pathology and for which instruments such a voice-related quality of life handicap index may be less applicable. Perhaps the adoption of a recently validated Transgender Voice Quality (applied in female-to-male transgendered patients) may permit for more clinically useful outcomes data sets.[24]

Interestingly, one study found that in female-to-male transgendered patients treated with testosterone, the sole predictor of satisfaction was the difference in frequency from pretreatment rather than the absolute posttreatment F_0.[25]

FUTURE DIRECTIONS

Fundamentally, the frequency of a vibrating structure is proportional to its tension and inversely proportional to its density. As such, in addition to procedures and speech therapy techniques to decrease vocal fold tension, there have been suggestions that interventions aimed at increasing vocal fold density may be of utility in pitch reduction procedures. An example would be vocal fold augmentation injection using a biocompatible material as favored by the author. Medialization laryngoplasty with infraglottic implant placement has also been suggested in well selected individuals.[26]

SUMMARY

Testosterone masculinizing hormone therapy in combination with speech retraining is effective in most of the male transgendered patients in deepening the voice to or near those of cisgendered men; however, a percentage fail to achieve a sufficiently masculine voice. In these patients, one of the three described pitch-lowering laryngeal framework procedures may be a safe and effective option. These techniques have also been used beneficially in other high-pitched voice disorders in cisgendered men and may play a role in nonbinary, gender-neutral and other individuals who seek a more masculine voice.

CLINICS CARE POINTS

- First line therapy for female to male transgendered patients should be an adequate trial of testosterone hormone therapy.
- First line therapy for mutational and other high-pitched voice disorders in cisgendered males is speech therapy.
- Surgical intervention for those who fail first line therapy is safe, and effective in experienced hands, with several different options and variations available in well-chosen patients.

DISCLOSURE

No financial or conflicts of interest to disclose.

REFERENCES

1. Hodges-Simeon CR, Grail GPO, Albert G, et al. Testosterone therapy masculinizes speech and gender presentation in transgender men. Sci Rep 2021;11(1): 3494.
2. McNeill EJ. Management of the transgender voice. J Laryngol Otol 2006;120(7): 521–3.
3. Dacakis G, Oates J, Douglas J. Beyond voice: perceptions of gender in male-to-female transsexuals. Curr Opin Otolaryngol Head Neck Surg 2012;20(3):165–70.
4. Gelfer MP, Bennett QE. Speaking fundamental frequency and vowel formant frequencies: effects on perception of gender. J Voice 2013;27(5):556–66.
5. Hillenbrand JM, Clark MJ. The role of f (0) and formant frequencies in distinguishing the voices of men and women. Atten Percept Psychophys 2009;71(5):1150–66.
6. Buckley DP, Dahl KL, Cler GJ, et al. Transmasculine voice modification: a case study. J Voice 2020;34(6):903–10.
7. Zamponi V, Mazzilli R, Mazzilli F, et al. Effect of sex hormones on human voice physiology: from childhood to senescence. Hormones 2021;20(4):691–6.
8. Hembree WC, Cohen-Kettenis PT, Gooren L, et al. Endocrine treatment of gender-dysphoric/gender-incongruent persons: an endocrine society clinical practice guideline. J Clin Endocrinol Metab 2017;102(11):3869–903.

9. Irwig MS, Childs K, Hancock AB. Effects of testosterone on the transgender male voice. Andrology 2017;5(1):107–12.
10. Azul D. Transmasculine people's vocal situations: a critical review of gender-related discourses and empirical data. Int J Lang Commun Disord 2015;50(1): 31–47.
11. Ziegler A, Henke T, Wiedrick J, et al. Effectiveness of testosterone therapy for masculinizing voice in transgender patients: a meta-analytic review. Int J Transgender 2019;19(1):25–45.
12. Cosyns M, Van Borsel J, Wierckx K, et al. Voice in female-to-male transsexual persons after long-term androgen therapy. Laryngoscope 2014;124(6):1409–14.
13. Isshiki N, Morita H, Okamura H, et al. Thyroplasty as a new phonosurgical technique. Acta Otolaryngol 1974;78(5–6):451–7.
14. Friedrich G, de Jong FI, Mahieu HF, et al. Laryngeal framework surgery: a proposal for classification and nomenclature by the Phonosurgery Committee of the European Laryngological Society. Eur Arch Otorhinolaryngol 2001;258(8): 389–96.
15. Bultynck C, Cosyns M, T'Sjoen G, et al. Thyroplasty type III to LOWER THE PITCH IN TRANS Men. Otolaryngol Head Neck Surg 2021;164(1):157–9.
16. Niimi S, Takemoto K, Shidara T. A surgical method for sulcus vocalis. Jap Otol (Toyko) 1973;76(Suppl):43.
17. Kocak I, Dogan M, Tadihan E, et al. Window anterior commissure relaxation laryngoplasty in the management of high-pitched voice disorders. Arch Otolaryngol Head Neck Surg 2008;134(12):1263–9.
18. Li GD, Mu L, Yang S. Acoustic evaluation of Isshiki type III thyroplasty for treatment of mutational voice disorders. J Laryngol Otol 1999;113(1):31–4.
19. Slavit DH, Maragos NE, Lipton RJ. Physiologic assessment of Isshiki tyle III thyroplasty. Laryngoscope 1990;100(8):844–8.
20. Hardy TLD, Boliek CA, Aalto D, et al. Contributions of voice and nonverbal communication to perceived masculinity-femininity for cisgender and transgender communicators. J Speech Lang Hear Res 2020;63(4):931–47.
21. Isshiki N, Taira T, Tanabe M. Surgical alteration of the vocal pitch. J Otolaryngol 1983;12(5):335–40.
22. Tucker HM. Anterior commissure laryngoplasty for adjustment of vocal fold tension. Ann Otol Rhinol Laryngol 1985;94(6 Pt 1):547–9.
23. Lennon CJ, Murry T, Sulica L. Vocal fold hemorrhage: factors predicting recurrence. Laryngoscope 2014;124(1):227–32.
24. Quinn S, Oates J, Dacakis G. Perceived gender and client satisfaction in transgender voice work: comparing self and listener rating scales across a training program. Folia Phoniatr Logop 2021. https://doi.org/10.1159/000521226.
25. Deuster D, Di Vincenzo K, Szukaj M, et al. Change of speech fundamental frequency explains the satisfaction with voice in response to testosterone therapy in female-to-male gender dysphoric individuals. Eur Arch Otorhinolaryngol 2016;273(8):2127–31.
26. Hoffman MR, Devine EE, Remacle M, et al. Combined type IIIB with bilateral type I thyroplasty for pitch lowering with maintenance of vocal fold tension. Eur Arch Otorhinolaryngol 2014;271(6):1621–9.

Opportunities for Gender-Affirming Surgery Training in Residency and Fellowship

Brian A. Nuyen, MD*, James P. Thomas, MD

KEYWORDS

- Otolaryngology • Residency training • Gender-affirming surgery
- Graduate medical education • Surgical education

KEY POINTS

- There are currently no national guidelines for gender-affirming care training standards for otolaryngology-head and neck surgery (OHNS).
- The most recent surveys of OHNS residents and program directors demonstrate limited availability of didactic and clinical training opportunities for gender-affirmation care, lower than analogous plastic surgery and urology resident reports. Available education is widely variable in content.
- Subspecialized training opportunities for residents and particularly fellows in facial and vocal gender affirmation surgical care exist in the United States with dedicated teaching and mentorship.

INTRODUCTION

Clinical understanding of head and neck anatomy, structure, and function are integral parts of otolaryngology-head and neck surgery training. This expertise afforded by otolaryngology-head and neck surgical education can translate into important opportunities to serve transgender and gender-nonconforming (TNG) communities. These specific training opportunities to be the best possible clinician and surgeon for TNG patients are becoming increasingly prevalent.

As the other articles in this textbook demonstrate, caring for the TNG patient in an OHNS clinic benefits from the specific understanding of complex interdisciplinary needs that transcend head and neck anatomy and pathophysiology. The surgeon must understand intrinsic concepts of gender, extrinsic gender perception manifestation in the head and neck, and understand the historical contextual relationships surgeons have with the TNG community. Most fundamentally, being able to heartfully

Dr J. P. Thomas and Dr B. A. Nuyen have no commercial or financial conflicts of interest and have no external funding sources for the work presented and discussed in this article.
Voice Doctor Clinic, 909 Northwest 18th Avenue, Portland, OR 97209, USA
* Corresponding author.
E-mail address: ba.nuyen@gmail.com

connect with TNG patients to elicit their honest concerns can make for an incredibly rewarding care experience for the patient and physician.

In this article here, we will discuss the limited but illuminating published literature describing OHNS training available in the care for the TNG patient, including gender-affirmation surgical training. Additionally, we will dive deeper into select interview conversations with current OHNS, facial plastics, and laryngology program and fellowship directors for their qualitative perspectives on OHNS gender-affirmation education.

THE NATIONAL LANDSCAPE OF HEAD AND NECK GENDER-AFFIRMATION SURGICAL TRAINING: SURVEY PERSPECTIVES FROM OTOLARYNGOLOGY-HEAD AND NECK SURGERY TRAINEES

Massenburg and colleagues in 2018 sought to shed light from a trainee perspective on the national landscape of head and neck gender-affirmation surgical training. They published a key study using validated cross-sectional surveys examining the current state of OHNS graduate medical education related to transgender patient care across the United States.[1]

A total 281 otolaryngology-head and neck surgery residents or fellows (68% of survey sent) participated in the survey, with all national regions obtaining greater than 65% response rate, with roughly even distribution of response across postgraduate year (PGY) 1 to 5 years, with twice as many male-identified survey respondents as female-identified.[1]

Eighty-three respondents (30% of the cohort) reported any/some kind of exposure to transgender patient care training. The West was the region with the highest proportion of respondents endorsing exposure. The authors in their surveys distinguished exposure between didactic educational experiences and clinical/direct patient care experiences. Within this cohort of respondents who endorsed exposure, didactic and patient care educational experiences within training were primarily focused on transgender surgical care, less so on medical and psychiatric-specific training.[1]

Exposure to transgender patient care training specifically in the form of head and neck gender-affirmation surgery was most commonly reported within feminizing or masculinizing facial surgery (55 respondents) and pitch alteration surgeries in the form of cricothyroid approximation or endoscopic shortening (52 respondents), and surgical management of complications of gender-affirming surgery (21 respondents). There were no apparent differences between men and women trainees in their reported types of exposure to surgical training.[1]

Opinions regarding the importance of gender-affirming surgery among OHNS trainees were also captured. Female-identified trainees ranked the importance higher on a Likert-scale than male-identified trainees. Trainees from the South and Midwest ranked the importance of gender-affirming surgical care lower compared with those from the Northeast. However, trainees from Northeast and West regions did not differ between each other in statistical significance in their overall high ranking of the importance of such care. PGY1s (those starting residency in June 2016) rated the importance of gender-affirming surgical care the highest compared with their other PGY counterparts.[1]

This was the first national representative study evaluating in a cross-sectional manner the quantified surveyed perspectives of OHNS trainees' exposure to transgender patient care and attitudes toward gender-affirming surgery.[1]

As of this article's publication, there are no educational competencies related to TNG care mandated by the Accreditation Council for Graduate Medical Education (ACGME)

Review committee for otolaryngology-head and neck surgery.[2] With the lack of mandated educational competencies, it is perhaps not surprising that only a minority of OHNS trainees (30%) reported any/some exposure to TNG health-care education. However, it is particularly noteworthy that the rates of exposure of this OHNS surveyed trainee cohort (30%) were lower than those reported by plastic surgery trainees (64%) and urology trainees (54%).[3–5] It highlights potential cultural differences across those academic training fields in prioritizing and emphasizing TNG care needs within those specialties. The authors of the study acknowledge that otolaryngologists are uniquely positioned with their knowledge of the head and neck to address critical TNG patient community needs.[1] Notably, there have been calls to action for greater OHNS training in TNG health care, including with head and neck gender affirmation surgery.[2,6–8]

The results of the surveyed OHNS trainee attitudes were also intriguing, as trainee attitudes toward the significance of the TNG care may reflect on the future of that care's provision. That female-identified trainees rated the importance of gender-affirming care higher than male-identified trainees was not surprising to the authors based on prior literature, in that female-identified individuals have previously demonstrated higher tolerance of LGBT communities.[9] Institutions in Northeast and Western regions may feature trainees friendlier to TNG communities given that those regions reflect a populace historically more in favor of TNG sociopolitical protections.[10] Most promisingly, the PGY1s (resident class in that study that started their residency training in 2016) had the highest ratings of the importance of gender-affirming surgery, perhaps signaling that the future of the field will invest more in the research, education, and clinical advocacy of TNG patient needs.

REPORTS FROM OTOLARYNGOLOGY-HEAD AND NECK SURGERY ACADEMIC TRAINING LEADERS: NATIONAL SURVEYS ON THE SEXUAL AND GENDER MINORITY TRAINING OPPORTUNITIES

Recently, Goetz and colleagues 2021 published a study examining sexual and gender minority curricula including TNG health-care education within otolaryngology residency programs. An adapted and validated survey was emailed to 116 OHNS residency program directors (112 Electronic Residency Application Service, 4 military) July through September 2019. A total of 65 complete responses (56% survey completion rate) were collected.[8]

The results demonstrated low overall offerings with large variability of didactic and clinical curricula offered. Mean percentage of total curriculum hours for sexual and gender minority topics was 1.0% for didactics and 0.7% for clinical exposure among those surveyed. Just less than half (42%) taught some aspect of informed sexual and gender minority care, which included proper pronoun usage, a sexual and gender minority care-specific history and physical, and intersectionality of identities. Half of programs featured education on facial gender-affirming procedures, and approximately half reported discussed vocal effects of gender-affirming hormone treatment (48%).[8]

In terms of program director attitudes, most program directors rated their perceived importance of OHNS training in sexual and gender minority care as "of average importance," "very important," or "absolutely essential." The authors found that such attitudes of importance were related to program directors' plans to increase sexual and gender minority-related residency education.[8]

The surveys also included results on plans and barriers to include competent training. When describing plans to include education, only 25% of program directors definitively endorsed intention to increase sexual and gender minority-related residency education. The majority believed that didactic lectures with visiting experts

(66%), followed by small group discussion (39%), and online modules (27%) were "best" formats to increase curricular content. The most common content areas of intended curriculum expansion during the next 3 years include facial gender-affirming procedures (19%) and managing facial changes associated with gender-affirming hormone treatment (12%). The most common reported barriers to including such training were lack of experienced faculty (52%) and lack of time (42%).[8]

Transgender/Nonbinary Care Training Opportunities Thoughts from Select Academic Training Leaders

Massenburg and colleagues[1] in 2018 and Goetz and colleagues[8] in 2021 showed with their quantitative data from cross-sectional validated surveys what the national landscape of TNG care education and gender-affirming care looked like. To investigate more deeply into facial and vocal gender-affirmation subspecialty training programs, the authors of this article spoke with select OHNS academic training leaders in facial and vocal gender-affirmation care for TNG patients. The authors interviewed definitively do not represent all available training opportunities in the United States but offer a unique array of qualitative and narrative perspectives.

In conversations with Dr Jeffrey Spiegel (he/him), Professor of Otolaryngology-Head and Neck Surgery at Boston University Medical Center and Director of The Spiegel Center in Newton, Massachusetts, article authors learned that Dr Spiegel has taught gender-affirming facial plastic and reconstructive surgery to OHNS residents since 2005 and facial plastic and reconstructive surgery (FPRS) fellows since the inception of his FPRS fellowship in 2009. Dr Spiegel's current caseload of facial feminization is about 5 cases a week. Otolaryngology PGY5 residents at Boston University Medical Center's OHNS residency program currently spend a 4 month block learning with him, with an approximately 60%/40% operating room/clinic split. Trainees are expected to learn how to properly greet and treat TNG patients and learn about the diverse ways TNG patients seek to affirm their gender in the head and neck. Such trainees also at the end of their training experience with him learn to understand facial gender perception and perioperative TNG care. Fellows of Dr Spiegel's program spend 70% of their fellowship with him personally and 30% of their fellowship with other attendings and educational pursuits, with a 50%/50% operating room/clinic split. One rewarding aspect he experiences as a teacher and mentor to his residents and fellows is how his trainees "learn to broaden their perspective on how to think about the face and appearance."

Article authors spoke with Dr Charles Shih (he/him), facial plastic/head and neck surgeon with Kaiser Permanente Northern California, who shared with article authors about the Kaiser Northern California OHNS residency experience in head and neck gender affirmation care, which started in 2016. Dr Shih noted that clinical training with TNG patients in facial gender-affirmation surgery runs throughout the PGY years, with graduated responsibility on individual and PGY learning level. Chief residents within the program embark upon "mini-fellowships" with goals for autonomous surgical care with multiple levels of attending support. Kaiser Northern California residents learn by participating in 1 to 2 surgical cases a week, among the faculty who have a combined caseload of running a facial gender affirmation operating room 5 times a week. Dr Shih said that he is proudest about his residents "having a unique exposure to an important yet marginalized patient population, an exposure that teaches the residents about their complex needs."

Dr Michael Nuara (he/him) spoke with the authors about his Virginia Mason Medical Center's facial gender affirmation experience in Seattle, Washington, which has provided training for the University of Washington (UW) OHNS residency and the UW

FPRS fellowship, now with its own separate dedicated FPRS fellowship that started in 2020. Facial gender affirmation surgical volume at Virginia Mason has accelerated significantly, previously one consultation a month to now one surgical case a week. Residents spend 2 months in their fourth year learning how to first assist in all aspects of the procedure, prioritizing involvement in rhinoplasty as a key indicator case. The Virginia Mason FPRS fellow is a key part of the gender affirmation facial plastics clinic and has an "intense" experience in surgical training, often primary surgeon for many cases. Dr Nuara is proudest of his training experience's "individualized and pragmatic approach," focused on cost-based reductions in quality facial feminization care. He enjoys training his residents and fellows in clinic, teaching them how to interact with someone who is gender nonconforming—"to me, that is where a lot of the education is."

Dr Rahul Seth (he/him) is an Associate Professor in the Division of Facial Plastic and Aesthetic Surgery at the University of California, San Francisco (UCSF), and codirector of the FPRS fellowship there, alongside Dr P. Daniel Knott. The UCSF facial plastics trainee team consists of a PGY3 or PGY5 resident with the UCSF FPRS fellow, participating in approximately 5 to 10 gender-affirming surgical cases a month. Surgical training emphasizes surgical decision-making, perioperative process including the informed consent procedures, facial plastic and reconstructive access to the whole face, and "unique and creative" problem-solving skills. Dr Seth noted that volume and specialized training with an FPRS fellowship is key to confidently launching a successful facial gender affirmation surgical practice. To Dr Seth, one of the most important things is that "residents and fellows gain exposure to understanding the challenges that transgender and nonbinary patients have in their lives and in their journeys. In the clinic and operating room, one of the things that is really notable and we try to stress are the journeys." Additionally, Dr Seth comments, "residents and fellows are taught an important lesson–how lifesaving these procedures are." Dr Seth also mentioned that he works closely with his UCSF Division of Laryngology colleagues, led by Dr Clark Rosen, for a multidisciplinary head and neck gender affirmation treatment panel.

Dr Joshua Rosenberg (he/him) is a facial plastic and reconstructive surgeon and Assistant Professor at Icahn School of Medicine and trains resident and fellows in facial gender-affirming care within Mount Sinai's Center for Transgender Medicine and Surgery. Dr Rosenberg commented that Mount Sinai has a largely "progressive and advanced" look at gender affirming care, with a centralized program with high priority assignment from hospital and academic medical center executive administration. OHNS residents in their PGY4 and PGY5 FPRS rotations participate in clinic and operating room opportunities. Dr Rosenberg's key learning objectives in the curriculum include trainees understanding "unconscious signifiers of masculine and feminine facial appearance" through didactic literature-based discussions and direct patient care experiences. With the Mount Sinai FRPS fellowship caseload experience of facial gender affirmation surgery often ranging between 20 and 40 per year, Dr Rosenberg expects his fellows to graduate proficient and competent in the full spectrum of the diverse procedures involved in facial feminization.

Dr Mark Courey (he/him), Professor of Otolaryngology-Head and Neck Surgery, Division Chief of Laryngology and Vice Chair of Quality for the Department of Otolaryngology-Head and Neck Surgery, and Director of the Grabscheid Voice and Swallowing Center at the Mount Sinai Health System is also part of Mount Sinai's Center for Transgender Medicine and Surgery. He clinically sees about 8 new TNG patients a week for vocal health concerns and works closely with speech language pathologists to help accomplish patient goals. He performs about 2 to 3 gender-affirming voice surgeries a week, primarily with Wendler glottoplasty techniques.[11] The laryngology service rotation at Mount Sinai occurs during residents' PGY4 year, with 1 month in laryngology clinic and OR, performing cases based on graduated responsibility. Mount Sinai laryngology fellows train 6 months exclusively with Dr Courey and participate in surgeries with him in a graduated manner as well. Dr Courey stated, "before the last couple of years, [such vocal surgeries] were not on the radar of these patients. We have since shown that we can have consistent results from surgery. I hope we are providing as a team of laryngologists and speech-language pathologists new avenues of treatment." Dr Courey added, "vocal gender-affirmation care allows me as a surgeon to teach about body theory, source filter theory, and bring it all together with surgery. We have to understand vocal science, behavioral skills, and surgical skills, and by breaking it down, it allows the trainee to focus on everything related to voice production."

Dr James Thomas (he/him), Medical Director of The Voice Doctor Clinic and Fellowship Director of his eponymous Laryngology Fellowship based in Portland, Oregon, has been providing vocal gender-affirming care since 2003. A pioneer of feminization laryngoplasty with thyrohyoid elevation[12,13] (additionally, see James P. Thomas' article, "Feminization Laryngoplasty"), Dr Thomas performs about 6 to 8 cases a month with his fellow, with graduated responsibility as the fellow progresses. Perioperative care is also emphasized, with postoperative follow-up care and long-term critical outcome assessment an important part of the fellowship experience. In addition to feminization laryngoplasty with thyrohyoid elevation, Dr Thomas also performs vocal webbing, feminizing chondrolaryngoplasty, adjunctive in-office and intraoperative laser reduction glottoplasty, and endoscopic vocal fold masculinization procedures as well. Dr Thomas described this private practice-academic fellowship as "a deep immersion in laryngology as a study of voice and physics of sound." An acoustic perspective with an emphasis on observant listening is the fellowship's foundation to gender laryngology in the training process, per Dr Thomas.

DISCUSSION

Massenburg and colleagues[1] 2018 and Goetz and colleagues[8] 2021 are important quantitative investigations in the national OHNS landscape of TNG care education and gender-affirming surgical training with their cross-sectional validated survey study design. They both revealed distinct themes of limited availability and varied representation of what that training looked like. Importantly, compared with plastic surgery and urology residents, otolaryngology residents have lower exposures to TNG care training.[3–5] However, younger trainees believed more strongly compared with older trainees about the importance of gender-affirming care, suggesting a promising future of otolaryngologists invested in TNG patient communities.[1] Goetz and colleagues in 2021 showed that almost 1 in 5 surveyed program directors had no explicit TNG patient care training at all during residency. However, most program directors believed sexual and gender minority health training including gender-affirmation care was of average importance, very important, or absolutely essential to their curricula.[8]

Narrative interviews looking more deeply into existing specialized training opportunities with select OHNS academic training leaders were particularly revealing. All interviewed academic directors, most of whom trained both residents and fellows, believed that all otolaryngology trainees, regardless of their plans to incorporate head and neck gender affirming care in their future practice, should master proper address including names and pronouns of TNG patients and be competent in comfortably establishing rapport with the TNG patient community with contextual respect to their historical and present-day marginalization. Dr Courey mentioned, "the understanding of the past and current trauma that these patients go through can make you a truly empathetic provider." Dr Nuara noted that otolaryngologists who do not perform gender-affirming procedures should still confidently and competently welcome and treat TNG patients in their practice, who will present with head and neck pathologic conditions outside of gender-affirmation concerns. Dr Shih commented that general otolaryngologists who have exposure to head and neck gender affirmation during their training are especially empowered to educate patients before they make the subspecialty referral; he notes that surgical and anatomic understanding of such techniques can help them help patients who may present acutely with surgical complications from such specialized procedures. Dr Courey and Dr Thomas each shared how training in vocal gender-affirmation care leads to more complex and nuanced understanding of the physics, acoustics, and other multidimensional properties of human voice. Almost all academic directors commented that OHNS trainees who ultimately do not perform head and neck gender affirmation in their careers but still were exposed to such training can still learn immensely from the surgical lessons, enhancing their ability to help all patients with head and neck trauma, cancer, complex inflammatory conditions, and cranial nerve pathologic condition.

The future directions of opportunities related to TNG care within otolaryngology-head and neck surgery are manifold. Dr Shih noted that while OHNS graduate medical education in gender affirming care is not currently widespread, he expects it to grow significantly in the next 10 years as newer generations of otolaryngology surgical trainees and teachers emerge amidst cultural and sociopolitical progression in TNG community protections. In Dr Seth's experience, he has noticed multiple calls to education in the field, and that OHNS trainees, in general, seek to learn more about head and neck gender affirmation but nationally do not receive enough training. Dr Nuara commented that OHNS gender-affirmation graduate medical education is often concentrated in major coastal cities in the United States with certain large swaths of the United States uncovered. He notes that ultimately social determinants of health and health-care training are intimately tied with voter and legislative decision-making, which has real current and future consequences for trainees and ultimately patients. Dr Rosenberg raised important emerging controversial questions regarding surgical procedure credentialing and certification, casting light on important issues related to protecting patient safety with quality care determinants but balancing access and reducing concerns for gatekeeping when such communities are already underserved.

Almost all academic directors explicitly mentioned that head and neck gender affirming care training was an endeavor OHNS academic departments needed to support. Dr Seth mentioned, "I think gender affirming facial surgery is uniquely positioned for the otolaryngologist to excel at. The changes to the face, due to our understanding of function and aesthetics–we are naturally attuned to the changes to the face. It's a calling that our specialty should answer to." The laryngologists interviewed agreed that laryngologists performing vocal gender-affirming surgery have a distinctively valuable skill set within multidisciplinary TNG care. Additionally, elective time so that residents could study with surgeons outside their institutions who currently perform these times of surgeries could be key.

SUMMARY

The national OHNS landscape of TNG care education and gender-affirming surgical training is variable with limited availability. However, specialized and innovative training with breadth and depth is available at select training sites focusing on facial and/or vocal gender affirmation throughout the United States. With growing trainee interest, motivated program and fellowship director-related efforts to expand training, and progressive arcs of social change focusing on protections and promotion of TNG health, the future of OHNS training opportunities to serve TNG patients is promising.

CLINICS CARE POINTS

- There are currently no national guidelines for gender-affirming care training standards for otolaryngology-head and neck surgery (OHNS).

- The most recent surveys of OHNS residents and program directors demonstrate limited availability of didactic and clinical training opportunities for gender-affirmation care, lower than analogous plastic surgery and urology resident reports. Available education is widely variable in content.

- Subspecialized training opportunities for residents and particularly fellows in facial and vocal gender affirmation surgical care exist in the United States with dedicated teaching and mentorship.

REFERENCES

1. Massenburg BB, Morrison SD, Rashidi V, et al. Educational exposure to transgender patient care in otolaryngology training. J Craniofac Surg 2018;29(5):1252–7.
2. Pregnall AM, Churchwell AL, Ehrenfeld JM. A call for LGBTQ content in graduate medical education program requirements. Acad Med 2021;96(6):828–35.
3. Dy GW, Osbun NC, Morrison SD, et al. Exposure to and attitudes regarding transgender education among urology residents. J Sex Med 2016;13:1466–72.
4. Morrison SD, Chong HJ, Dy GW, et al. Educational exposure to transgender patient care in plastic surgery training. Plast Reconstr Surg 2016;138:944–53.
5. Morrison SD, Dy GW, Chong HJ, et al. Transgender-related education in plastic surgery and urology residency programs. J Grad Med Educ 2017;9:178–83.
6. Pasternak K, Francis DO. An update on treatment of voice-gender incongruence by otolaryngologists and speech-language pathologists. Curr Opin Otolaryngol Head Neck Surg 2019;27(6):475–81.
7. Juszczak HM, Fridirici Z, Knott PD, et al. An update in facial gender confirming surgery. Curr Opin Otolaryngol Head Neck Surg 2019;27(4):243–52.
8. Goetz TG, Nieman CL, Chaiet SR, et al. Sexual and gender minority curriculum within otolaryngology residency programs. Transgend Health 2021;6(5):267–74.
9. Holland L, Matthews TL, Schott MR. That's so gay!" Exploring college students' attitudes toward the LGBT population. J Homosex 2013;60:575–95.
10. James, S E., Herman, J, Keisling, M, et al. 2015 U.S. Transgender survey (USTS). Inter-university consortium for political and social research [distributor], 2019-05-22. https://doi.org/10.3886/ICPSR37229.v1
11. Chang J, Brown SK, Hu S, et al. Effect of wendler glottoplasty on acoustic measures of voice. Laryngoscope 2021;131(3):583–6.
12. Thomas JP, MacMillan C. Feminization laryngoplasty: assessment of surgical pitch elevation. Eur Arch Otorhinolaryngol 2013;270(10):2695–700.
13. Nuyen BA, Qian ZJ, Campbell RD, et al. Feminization laryngoplasty: 17-year review on long-term outcomes, safety, and technique. Otolaryngol Head Neck Surg 2021. 01945998211036870.

Sex-Related Characteristics of the Face

Arushi Gulati, BS, P. Daniel Knott, MD, Rahul Seth, MD*

KEYWORDS

- Gender • Facial analysis • Facial sex characteristics • Facial feminization surgery
- Facial masculinization surgery

KEY POINTS

- Structural and volumetric differences exist between the male and female face from birth but morphology becomes more differentiated at puberty.
- A horizontal-thirds framework can be used to guide analysis of gender presentation and facial features relative to ideal measurements and patient-specific goals.
- The male face is longer, wider, and more rectangular and is characterized by brow prominence. The female face is more rounded and has less angulated features, although specific differences vary by age and ethnicity.

BACKGROUND

The human face and neck are central to individual identity and are among the first physical aspects to be noted by others during social encounters. Facial appearance, including size and shape, is highly variable among individuals and consists of a complex layered arrangement of bone, muscle, fat, and skin. This overall structure is influenced by a multitude of factors, including genetics, race, ethnicity, age, and sex.[1-3]

Facial appearance plays a key role in subconscious recognition and encoding of gender identity based on the presence of recognizable sexual dimorphisms in facial structure. Although some studies have provided evidence of sex-based differences in the neurocranial size and facial structure of infants, gender-based distinctions in the neonatal and early childhood periods are extremely subtle.[4-6] Instead, expression of sex-typical facial traits is driven by the production of hormones typically associated with the onset of puberty. Increased testosterone levels trigger masculinization around 13 years of age.[4]

Gender-specific facial characteristics vary broadly, from craniofacial structure to skin and soft tissue distribution. Advancements in photogrammetry, laser scanning

Division of Facial Plastic and Reconstructive Surgery, Department of Otolaryngology- Head and Neck Surgery, University of California San Francisco, 2233 Post Street, 3rd Floor, San Francisco, CA 94115, USA
* Corresponding author.
E-mail address: rahul.seth@ucsf.edu

Otolaryngol Clin N Am 55 (2022) 775–783
https://doi.org/10.1016/j.otc.2022.04.012
0030-6665/22/© 2022 Elsevier Inc. All rights reserved.

oto.theclinics.com

of 3-dimensional surfaces, and improved systems for medical imaging have allowed us to extract morphometric data that defines the relationship between facial landmarks and identifies variations between sexes.[7] For instance, the male face is longer, wider, and more rectangular with a flatter forehead than the female face, which is typically more rounded in structure and has a higher upper face.[8,9] Although overall data are mixed, some studies have also demonstrated a correlation between degree of sexual dimorphism and perceived attractiveness. This may be due to evolutionary selection for dominant behavior in men or may be related to signaling of underlying health during mate selection.[10–13]

Although surgical techniques aimed at altering facial gender identity in transgender and gender-diverse individuals have been extensively described in the surgical literature, relative contribution of specific differences in facial shape and form to overall sexual dimorphism have not yet been well described and are likely highly context-dependent.[9] Therefore, overall masculine or feminine appearance should be considered as a sum of multiple measurable differences in facial structure. Successful gender-affirming facial surgery requires a comprehensive understanding of these measures and mastery over the means to reliably alter the relevant structures. This article aims to provide a framework for identification and analysis of sex-based differences in facial anatomy that can be used to guide individualized approaches to surgical planning to create congruence with the patients' existing physical features and goals for gender expression.

APPROACH TO FACIAL ANALYSIS

A multitude of approaches has been advanced to facilitate facial analysis. The golden ratio (1.618) has been considered an esthetic ideal in architecture and natural forms since antiquity, although its correlation with attractiveness has not been consistently demonstrated.[14] More recently, the neoclassical canon of facial proportions was developed by Renaissance artists to divide artistic expressions of the face into symmetric vertical fifths and equal horizontal thirds.[15] Clinical practice has exposed the limits of this paradigm because wide differences occur across races and ethnicities. Additional esthetic ideals for comparison of faces, such as the use of the Frankfurt horizontal plane and Powell and Humphrey's esthetic angles, have also been developed.[14]

Given the prevalence of the horizontal-thirds framework in current surgical planning for gender-affirming facial surgery, the facial structure has been described here using the same divisions. Thus, discussion of skeletal and soft tissue differences between male and female facial anatomy has been divided into 3 main regions: (1) upper third, including the forehead and brow; (2) middle third, including the orbit, nose, and cheeks; and (3) lower third, including the lips, mandible, and chin.

UPPER FACE

The upper face extends from the trichion, superiorly, to the glabella, inferiorly. Evaluation of this region should include the hairline, forehead, glabella, and brow. Earlier study by Bruce and colleagues has demonstrated that masking of eyes in photographs produces a greater disruption to gender recognition than masking of the nose or mouth, and significant information may be obtained when the eyebrow is not masked.[16] Similarly, experiments by Brown and Perett have demonstrated that when features are presented in isolation, the brow and eyes provide the greatest amount of information in identifying gender.[17] Finally, in a study conducted by Spiegel, modification of the forehead of men in photographs was found to be more feminizing than middle-third or lower-third facial modification in both frontal and profile view.[18] Considering together, these studies suggest that the upper face is particularly important to gender determination. (**Fig. 1**)

Sexual dimorphism is apparent in both hairline shape and location. In women, the hairline is characterized by a rounded or rectangular, nonreceding pattern with a shorter distance from the midglabella to the trichion (mean 5.0–5.8 cm).[19,20] The male hairline is more likely M-shaped with temporal recessions and with a greater distance from the midglabella to the trichion (mean 6–8 cm) that may further increase with androgenic alopecia.[19–21] Men also tend to have greater temporal hollowing of the soft tissue of the hairline and forehead than women.[19]

Cephalometric measurements of the frontonasal-orbital complex additionally differ by sex and are a key instrument for sex determination in osteological collections.[2] In women, the frontal bone seems both more vertical and more rounded, creating a smooth convexity. The male frontal bone has more horizontal protrusion at the forehead and the supraorbital ridge, creating an inclined shape that is flatter and less steep than seen in women.[22,23] Additionally, the presence of a well-developed supraorbital ridge in men creates a curvature that is discontinuous with the upper forehead. This results in a projected glabella with a narrower nasofrontal angle. Given that the supraorbital ridge in women is relatively minimal, women conversely tend to have a relatively flat glabella with a wider nasofrontal angle.[15,24] One hypothesis for the presence of these skeletal differences is variation in frontal sinus pneumatization between the sexes.[25]

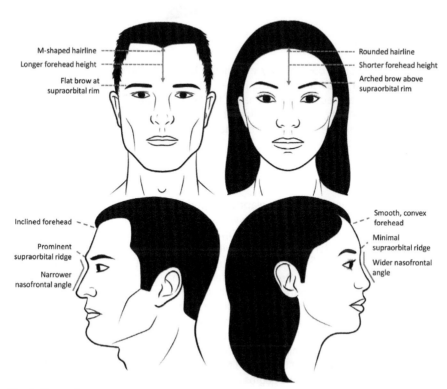

Fig. 1. Upper face.

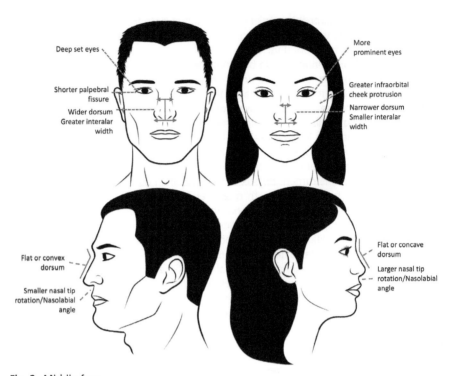

Deep set eyes

More prominent eyes

Shorter palpebral fissure

Greater infraorbital cheek protrusion

Wider dorsum
Greater interalar width

Narrower dorsum
Smaller interalar width

Flat or concave dorsum

Flat or convex dorsum

Larger nasal tip rotation/Nasolabial angle

Smaller nasal tip rotation/Nasolabial angle

Fig. 2. Middle face.

Eyebrows, although cosmetically modifiable based on individual preference, are typically straighter, heavier, and flatter in men. In contrast, the female brow is typically thinner and more arched, rising to a peak at the lateral limbus.[18] The male brow is also located more inferiorly, usually residing at the level of the supraorbital rim in men versus several millimeters above the supraorbital rim in women.[26]

MIDDLE FACE

The middle face extends from the glabella, superiorly, to the subnasale, inferiorly. In this region, consideration should be given to the orbits and periorbital tissue, nose, zygoma, and soft tissue of the cheeks. **(Fig. 2)**

Data comparing orbital size are mixed, with some studies describing a larger orbital height and width in men,[3,27,28] whereas others suggest that women typically have a larger orbital aperture.[7,19,22] Degree of difference may be additionally impacted by age and ethnicity.[27,28] Nevertheless, the male eyes seem more deeply set in relation to the facial plane with narrower palpebral fissures and a greater intercanthal distance, whereas female eyes seem more prominent, with a smaller intercanthal distance and higher relative location.[7,19] The presence of larger eyes in proportion to the face is associated with a more feminine appearance and a more attractive feminine face.[22]

Regarding periorbital soft tissue, the position of the supratarsal crease is typically lower in men than women, although the degree of difference is again dependent on ethnicity. In studies of white or Caucasian patients, the upper lid crease lies an average of 7 to 8 mm above the lid margin in men and 10 to 12 mm above the lid margin in women. The upper lid crease in Asian populations may be lower or absent.[29] There are no significant differences in the morphology of the lower eyelids between men and women.[15,29]

On frontal view, the male face is characterized by a long and wide nasal shape. In contrast, the female nose is both vertically and transversely smaller in size.[22] This is in part due to the presence of wider nasal bones with a steeper nasal inclination, a wider dorsum, and a higher nasion in men.[7,30] Additionally, the male nose has a wider nasal base with greater interalar width (3.5–3.8 cm) and minimal supratip break compared with the female nose (interalar width: 3.2–3.4 cm).[30–33]

Earlier study by Chronicle and colleagues suggest that profile or three-quarter views of the nose may play a greater role in gender identification than frontal views.[34] On profile view, the male nasofrontal angle is usually narrower due to greater glabellar projection, as described above, and the nasal tip is also more anteriorly projected than the female nasal tip by up to 5 mm.[19] The relatively wide nasofrontal angle and posterior nasal tip location in women creates a less protuberant profile and an overall softer appearance with a less abrupt transition between the forehead and nose. The male nose is also characterized by a flat or slightly convex shape (ie, a "dorsal hump"), although the female nose is more commonly associated with a narrow, concave dorsum, although exact nasal shape is again highly ethnicity-dependent.[30] Finally, the male nose has a smaller degree of nasal tip rotation, with a nasolabial angle of 100° to 103° in men versus 105° to 108° in women.[35]

The zygomatic arch is more pronounced in men, with a higher and more lateral site of maximal projection and greater extension inferiorly.[36] In contrast, women have a rounder arch with a more medial site of maximal projection. Despite the less prominent zygomatic arch, women typically have a greater infraorbital sagittal cheek protrusion accompanied by submalar hollowing that results in an accentuated appearance of the cheekbone.[7,15,22]

LOWER FACE

The lower face extends from the subnasale, superiorly to the chin, inferiorly. This region contains the lips, jaw, and chin, all of which play key roles in gender expression. The lower face height may be greater in men than women due to a vertically longer mandible.[22] (**Fig. 3**)

Although male lips have a greater thickness and total volume, the male labial morphology is characterized by a thin upper lip and a smaller upper-to-lower lip ratio.[37] Women, however, have a shorter transverse lip length and greater vertical height of the upper lip.[18] This increased height-to-width ratio in women provides the appearance of greater fullness. Female upper labial morphology is also characterized by a more angulated Cupid's bow and greater vermillion show.[15,37] The lower lip height–width ratio is similar between sexes.[37]

Although shape dimorphism may already exist in the mandible by birth, the growth rate during puberty is greater in men, resulting in a mandible that is larger in size with a more prominent angle, more elongated body, taller ramus, and lateral flaring with a greater inter-ramus distance.[38,39] Additionally, the mandibular height-to-width ratio is larger in men, and the chin and lower jaw may be up to 20% longer than in women.[15,22] The result is a more protruded and broader mandible in men that extends steeply downward before squaring off at the basal symphysis, creating a rectangular facial structure. In comparison, women tend to have a narrower and more rounded or pointed chin, creating a heart-shaped or inverted pyramid-shaped facial structure.[38,39] The larger mandibular size in men may be in part due to the presence of greater masseteric attachments, which additionally contribute to the wider

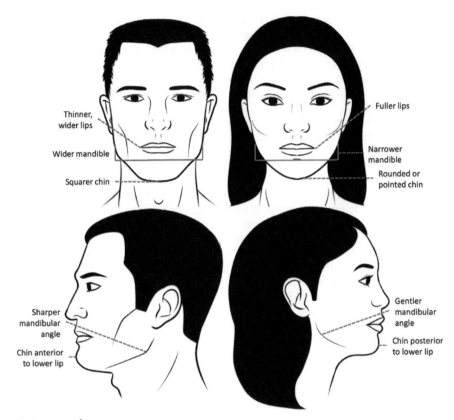

Thinner, wider lips

Fuller lips

Wider mandible

Narrower mandible

Squarer chin

Rounded or pointed chin

Sharper mandibular angle

Gentler mandibular angle

Chin anterior to lower lip

Chin posterior to lower lip

Fig. 3. Lower face.

appearance of the male jawline.[15] Finally, it is important to note that malocclusion of dental structures may affect an individual's cephalometric relationships within the lower third of the face.[15]

ADDITIONAL CONSIDERATIONS

It is important to note that characteristics described here represent overall trends and that both degree of difference in facial structure between sexes and esthetic ideals may vary by individual. Furthermore, facial structure may be modified by additional factors such as age and ethnicity.

For instance, facial features continue to change with aging because of cellular turnover, alterations in hormone levels, and environmental damage (eg, sun exposure) that result in skin thinning, fat redistribution, soft tissue descent, and bone resorption. Morphologic changes in the skull, such as widening of the cranium and retrusion of the forehead, reduce the accuracy of sex classification using bony features, with a trend toward masculinization in women.[2] Additionally, loss of osseous and ligamentous support for soft tissue and increased laxity of the skin causes descent of periorbital tissues, including the brow, further resulting in a masculinized appearance.[18]

Differences in facial proportions between ethnicities have been extensively demonstrated. Variations at nearly every level of the face, from orbital structure to nasal and labial shape greatly limit the generalizability of published ideal values.[1,28,29,40] Given that a large proportion of morphometric research has been conducted in white or Caucasian individuals, there is a need for ethnicity-specific normative values for guidance in surgical planning. However, given the heterogenous ethnic composition of most individuals, an approach that understands the normative corelation and codependence of facial features may be the optimum approach in facial analysis for gender-affirming surgery.[41] Thus, the structural differences described here are not prescriptive but rather meant to serve as a starting point to help surgeons consider how individual facial features can be used to better align a patient's gender identity and gender expression.

SUMMARY

There are several key differences in facial shape and form that differentiate the male and female facial silhouettes, from the craniofacial structure to skin and soft tissue distribution. Careful consideration to each of the facial thirds can provide surgeons with a framework to identify facial structures that may be altered to allow individuals to best express their gender identify. However, given strong interrelationships, structures must be judiciously altered relative to one another and in accordance with patient preferences to provide the desired degree of masculinity or femininity.

CLINICS CARE POINTS

- Structural and volumetric differences exist between the male and female face from birth but morphology becomes more differentiated at puberty and can be broadly categorized by differences in size and shape.

- The male face is longer, wider, and more rectangular with a prominent brow, whereas the female face is more rounded with less angulated features.

- As facial differences are partially age-dependent and ethnicity-dependent, these factors should be considered.

DISCLOSURE

The authors have no relevant conflicts of interest to disclose.

REFERENCES

1. Kleisner K, Tureček P, Roberts SC, et al. How and why patterns of sexual dimorphism in human faces vary across the world. Sci Rep 2021;11(1):5978.
2. Velemínská J, Fleischmannová N, Suchá B, et al. Age-related differences in cranial sexual dimorphism in contemporary Europe. Int J Legal Med 2021;135(5):2033–44.
3. Sforza C, Grandi G, Catti F, et al. Age- and sex-related changes in the soft tissues of the orbital region. Forensic Sci Int 2009;185(1):115.e1–8.
4. Matthews H, Penington T, Saey I, et al. Spatially dense morphometrics of craniofacial sexual dimorphism in 1-year-olds. J Anat 2016;229(4):549–59.
5. Kaminski G, Méary D, Mermillod M, et al. Is it a he or a she? behavioral and computational approaches to sex categorization. Atten Percept Psychophys 2011;73(5):1344–9.

6. Wild HA, Barrett SE, Spence MJ, et al. Recognition and sex categorization of adults' and children's faces: examining performance in the absence of sex-stereotyped cues. J Exp Child Psychol 2000;77(4):269–91.

7. Velemínská J, Bigoni L, Krajíček V, et al. Surface facial modelling and allometry in relation to sexual dimorphism. Homo 2012;63(2):81–93.

8. Ferrario VF, Sforza C, Pizzini G, et al. Sexual dimorphism in the human face assessed by euclidean distance matrix analysis. J Anat 1993;183(Pt 3):593–600.

9. Mydlová M, Dupej J, Koudelová J, et al. Sexual dimorphism of facial appearance in ageing human adults: a cross-sectional study. Forensic Sci Int 2015;257: 519.e1–9.

10. Nakamura K, Watanabe K. A new data-driven mathematical model dissociates attractiveness from sexual dimorphism of human faces. Sci Rep 2020;10:16588.

11. Penton-Voak IS, Jones BC, Little AC, et al. Symmetry, sexual dimorphism in facial proportions and male facial attractiveness. Proc Biol Sci 2001;268(1476): 1617–23.

12. Schaefer K, Fink B, Grammer K, et al. Female appearance: Facial and bodily attractiveness as shape. Psychol Sci 2006;48(2):187–204.

13. Mueller U, Mazur A. Facial dominance in homo sapiens as honest signaling of male quality. Behav Ecol 1997;8.

14. Prendergast P. Facial proportions. In: Advanced surgical facial rejuvenation: art and clinical practice. 2012. p. 15–22.

15. Lakhiani C, Somenek MT. Gender-related facial analysis. Facial Plast Surg Clin North Am 2019;27(2):171–7.

16. Bruce V, Burton AM, Hanna E, et al. Sex discrimination: how do we tell the difference between male and female faces? Perception 1993;22(2):131–52.

17. Brown E, Perrett DI. What gives a face its gender? Perception 1993;22(7):829–40.

18. Spiegel JH. Facial determinants of female gender and feminizing forehead cranioplasty. Laryngoscope 2011;121(2):250–61.

19. Dang BN, Hu AC, Bertrand AA, et al. Evaluation and treatment of facial feminization surgery: part I. forehead, orbits, eyebrows, eyes, and nose. Arch Plast Surg 2021;48(5):503–10.

20. Sirinturk S, Bagheri H, Govsa F, et al. Study of frontal hairline patterns for natural design and restoration. Surg Radiol Anat 2017;39(6):679–84.

21. Garcia-Rodriguez L, Thain LM, Spiegel JH. Scalp advancement for transgender women: closing the gap. Laryngoscope 2020;130(6):1431–5.

22. Tanikawa C, Zere E, Takada K. Sexual dimorphism in the facial morphology of adult humans: a three-dimensional analysis. PLoS One 2016;67(1):23–49.

23. Del Bove A, Profico A, Riga A, et al. A geometric morphometric approach to the study of sexual dimorphism in the modern human frontal bone. Am J Phys Anthropol 2020;173(4):643–54.

24. Garvin HM, Ruff CB. Sexual dimorphism in skeletal browridge and chin morphologies determined using a new quantitative method. Am J Phys Anthropol 2012; 147(4):661–70.

25. Ousterhout DK. Feminization of the forehead: contour changing to improve female aesthetics. Plast Reconstr Surg 1987;79(5):701–13.

26. Yalçınkaya E, Cingi C, Söken H, et al. Aesthetic analysis of the ideal eyebrow shape and position. Eur Arch Otorhinolaryngol 2016;273(2):305–10.

27. Ferrario VF, Sforza C, Colombo A, et al. Morphometry of the orbital region: a soft-tissue study from adolescence to mid-adulthood. Plast Reconstr Surg 2001; 108(2):285–92.

28. Ghorai L, Asha ML, Lekshmy J, et al. Orbital aperture morphometry in Indian population: a digital radiographic study. J Forensic Dent Sci 2017;9(2):61–4.
29. Most SP, Mobley SR, Larrabee WF. Anatomy of the eyelids. Facial Plast Surg Clin North Am 2005;13(4):487–92, v.
30. Springer IN, Zernial O, Nölke F, et al. Gender and nasal shape: measures for rhinoplasty. Plast Reconstr Surg 2008;121(2):629–37.
31. Miranda GA, D'Souza M. Evaluating the reliability of the interalar width and intercommissural width as guides in selection of artificial maxillary anterior teeth: a clinical study. J Interdiscip Dent 2016;6(2):64.
32. Smith BJ. The value of the nose width as an esthetic guide in prosthodontics. J Prosthet Dent 1975;34(5):562–73.
33. Deogade SC, Mantri SS, Sumathi K, et al. The relationship between innercanthal dimension and interalar width to the intercanine width of maxillary anterior teeth in central Indian population. J Indian Prosthodont Soc 2015;15(2):91–7.
34. Chronicle EP, Chan MY, Hawkings C, et al. You can tell by the nose–judging sex from an isolated facial feature. Perception 1995;24(8):969–73.
35. Bhat U, Peswani AR, Wagh S, et al. Optimising results of nasal tip rotation applying combination of nasolabial angle and lip–columellar angle in tandem in patients operated by "cock-up" alar cartilage flaps technique. Indian J Plast Surg 2019;52(2):183–94.
36. Schlager S, Rüdell A. Sexual dimorphism and population affinity in the human zygomatic structure—comparing surface to outline data. Anat Rec 2017;300(1):226–37.
37. Ferrario VF, Rosati R, Peretta R, et al. Labial morphology: a 3-dimensional anthropometric study. J Oral Maxillofac Surg 2009;67(9):1832–9.
38. Fan Y, Penington A, Kilpatrick N, et al. Quantification of mandibular sexual dimorphism during adolescence. J Anat 2019;234(5):709–17.
39. Coquerelle M, Bookstein FL, Braga J, et al. Sexual dimorphism of the human mandible and its association with dental development. Am J Phys Anthropol 2011;145(2):192–202.
40. Hwang HS, Kim WS, McNamara JA. Ethnic differences in the soft tissue profile of Korean and European-American adults with normal occlusions and well-balanced faces. Angle Orthod 2002;72(1):72–80.
41. Bannister JJ, Juszczak H, Aponte JD, et al. Sex differences in adult facial three-dimensional morphology: application to gender-affirming facial surgery. Facial Plast Surg Aesthet Med 2022. Epub ahead of print.

Brow Bossing Reduction

Bryan Rolfes, MD

KEYWORDS

- Brow bossing • Forehead reduction • Forehead feminization • FFS • GCFS

KEY POINTS

- The gender-defining features of the upper face.
- Approach to reshaping the hairline.
- Techniques to reduce brow bossing.
- Reshaping the orbital rims.

 Video content accompanies this article at http://www.oto.theclinics.com.

INTRODUCTION

For most of us, gender assessment is a split second, unconscious process that is based on multiple physical and social cues, and the default is a binary result. This assessment is unconsciously performed many times every day. Those gender cues can include mannerisms, dress, voice, and physical features. In most situations, it is physical features that have the most significant effect on the conclusion. Which physical features convey the most information in any gender assessment varies with the situation, but facial features tend to be the most significant in our most intimate interactions. While there are gender-specific variations in features throughout the face, some areas more powerfully confirm gender than others. Of the areas that confirm a masculine gender, the forehead is the most powerful.[1] That often makes the upper face the most significant source of gender dysphoria for many transfeminine individuals. Properly addressing this area is essential to achieve consistent patient satisfaction after gender-confirming facial surgery (GCFS). Over the past 40 years, surgical techniques have been developed and refined to reduce the masculine features of the forehead. In most patients, the shape and relative ratios of the forehead can be safely and consistently brought within an average feminine range.

Pinnacle Cosmetic, 935 Wayzata Boulevard E, Suite 200, Wayzata, MN 55391, USA
E-mail address: Bryan.Rolfes@PinnacleCosmetic.com

Otolaryngol Clin N Am 55 (2022) 785–795
https://doi.org/10.1016/j.otc.2022.04.003
0030-6665/22/© 2022 Elsevier Inc. All rights reserved.

oto.theclinics.com

HISTORY

Dr Doug Ousterhout is generally considered the founder of GCFS in the United States. He was the first to develop new and refine existing procedures specifically to treat gender dysphoria.

In his foundational article on feminizing the forehead in 1987, Ousterhout first examined thousands of skulls from an anthropology collection to determine gender-specific contour variations. Skulls of men tended to have more anterior projection of the brow and orbital rims with a flattened mid-forehead. The skulls of women had foreheads that were more vertical, while in men there was a posterior slope as you ascend toward the parietal bone. Ousterhout then divided patients who presented with masculine upper facial features into 3 groups based on their degree of brow bossing and the size and structure of their frontal sinus. The patient's group would determine their optimal treatment technique. Group 1 had moderate brow bossing and a hypoplastic frontal sinus with a thick anterior table. Optimal treatment of patients in this group involved a reductive burring of the bone of the brow and orbital rim. With the thick anterior table, adequate reduction could be achieved while still leaving enough bone to protect the frontal sinus from fracture. Group 2 had moderate brow bossing, a thick anterior table, and a flattened mid-forehead. Optimal treatment required reduction with burring with the addition of methyl methacrylate to augment and round the mid-forehead above the brow. Group 3 had significant brow bossing and a thin anterior table. Optimal treatment of this group required osteotomies around the border of and setback of the anterior table of the frontal sinus with reductive burring to contour the thicker bone of the lateral brow and orbital rims.[2] Ousterhout subsequently described a fourth group in whom the entire forehead was hypoplastic. There was no brow bossing, but the flattened mid-forehead created a masculine appearance. This group required no reduction, but the augmentation of the entire forehead with methyl methacrylate to create a more rounded shape and more vertical slope. The same basic principles are still used today.

GENDER-SPECIFIC VARIATIONS IN THE UPPER THIRD OF THE FACE

Exposure to testosterone creates changes in the facial structure and hair patterns that contribute to a masculine appearance. A feminine face is a face without masculine features. A single strong masculine feature can create a face that is consistently assigned a male gender, and the features that can most powerfully convey a masculine gender are in the upper one-third of the face.[1]

A masculine hairline is higher than a feminine hairline. The average hairline height measurement associated with each gender varies between ethnic groups, but within each group, the average height for a masculine hairline is higher than the average height for a feminine hairline. At least as important as height is the hairline shape. Testosterone creates characteristic patterns of recession giving a masculine hairline an "M" shape. A minority of feminine hairlines are also "M" shaped, but because the mature male hairline is rarely round the goal of surgery is to make the hairline as round as possible.[3]

Gender-specific variations in contour are present throughout the forehead. In a masculine upper forehead, the frontal eminences are more prominent creating a flattened central forehead plateau. The temporal ridge is more prominent creating a deeper, more concave temporal fossa.

A masculine lower forehead has a brow and orbital rims with a more anterior and inferior projection that creates a smaller, hooded orbit. This more projected brow makes the forehead slope back toward the hairline, while a feminine forehead is more vertical. The eyebrow itself is lower and flatter in shape compared with an age-matched feminine eyebrow.[1,4,5]

CREATING A MORE FEMININE HAIRLINE

The 2 primary methods used to change the hairline are hair grafting and surgical hairline advancement. Hair grafting can be either follicular unit extraction (FUE) or follicular unit transplantation (FUT). FUT is more commonly employed for gender confirmation as there is typically enough hair to cover the scar from the strip harvest and it is more cost-effective. Hair grafting is most often performed as a staged procedure but can be performed concurrently with a donor strip removed from the coronal incision line. This technique can result in good graft take when the proper facilities and staffing are in place.[6] When staged, hair grafting can be used to further lower and round the hairline after surgical advancement, and/or to disguise the hairline advancement scar.

To perform a surgical hairline advancement, a coronal incision is made that is 2 to 3 cm behind the hairline in the temples, but along the anterior hairline between the temporal tufts (henceforth referred to as a "hairline incision"). This incision leads to the most visible scar for most patients after a GCFS . To best disguise this scar, an irregular trichophytic technique should be used, especially in the central portion of the incision along the hairline. The irregularly irregular course of the incision will help the final hairline best match the variations seen in a presurgical hairline. Even when the incisional scar is not visible, a hairline without variation looks quite unnatural. A sharply beveled trichophytic incision will allow the transected hair shafts to regrow through the scar and even the lower skin flap itself. This technique is most effective when the hair shafts are angled toward the incision and are less productive over the temple where the shafts are typically angled parallel to the incision. Adequate hemostasis can be obtained in most patients with judicious cautery and wrapping the leading edge of the upper flap in laps. Cautery use should be targeted to avoid hair follicle loss. Raney clips are not necessary. Tissue elevation in the subgaleal plane is performed to the vertex. The galea is scored if maximal advancement is needed. These incisions should be short, discontinuous, and only through the galea to preserve the vascular network. Using these techniques, an average of 2 cm of advancement is achieved.[7] The hair-bearing flap is pulled over the lower forehead flap, and the overlap is marked. The portion of the lower flap that is superior to this mark can then be resected. Before making this incision consider what effect the width and shape of the resection will have on both the lowering of the hairline and the lifting of the brows to create the best location and shape for both. The use of bone anchors, a bioabsorbable fixation device, or sutures through monocortical tunnels can be used to reduce tension at the incision and may reduce scar width. These fixation methods can also be used to achieve better control of flap position to improve preexisting asymmetry of the hairline or eyebrows. A layered closure is then performed with good approximation of the galea. The temporal aspects of the lower flap are rotated medially to round the hairline and minimize the length of the incision along the hairline.

These techniques are often sufficient to round the hairline when early recession is present. In cases whereby the target hairline is not achieved, hair grafting is recommended. Visible scarring can be treated with scar revision or camouflaged with hair grafting at least 6 months after surgery when the scar has matured.[8]

When the hairline shape and height are already feminine, or if there is a history of unusually visible scarring, a coronal incision well into the hairline is used. When healed, this scar would only be visible after significant hair loss. Orchiectomy or hormone blockers will prevent androgenic alopecia. The patient should be counseled that their hairline will be slightly higher after surgery, as after bone reduction their soft tissue will need to be lifted to prevent brow ptosis.

CREATING A MORE FEMININE FOREHEAD CONTOUR

The chosen access incision, hairline versus coronal, is carried directly down through the periosteum. Caudal elevation is in the subperiosteal plane between the temporalis muscles to allow for contouring of the bone as needed. Laterally, subfascial elevation over the temporalis provides maximal frontal branch protection.[9] Care is used when elevating the more adherent periosteum over the superciliary arch until the supraorbital foramen is identified. Occasionally the supraorbital nerve travels in a groove on the caudal aspect of the excessively projected bone and is easily reflected and protected during removal. More often the nerve exits through a foramen and must be drilled out for an optimal result. Caudally, the periosteum should be elevated to the radix and over the orbital rim into the orbit. Laterally, the zygomaticofrontal suture should be exposed.

After tissue elevation, the contour of the bone is assessed and the areas to be reduced are marked. In the upper forehead, a powered rotary device is used to round the frontal bone, remove the frontal eminances, and reduce the temporal ridge. In the lower forehead, the anterior projection of the lateral orbital rims is first reduced to the desired level. Then this new contour is carried medially from each side until the frontal sinus is encountered. The point where reducing the brow to the desired level of projection meets the frontal sinus is found and followed around the perimeter of the sinus. It is difficult to further reduce the brow projection with a second pass using this method, as the anterior table will then be too small to fit the defect. The perimeter is "blue lined," typically with a diamond burr to avoid stripping the mucosa from areas of the simus. A circumferential sinusotomy is made with an osteotome or saw where needed, and the bone island is carefully removed. The mucosa is elevated from any visible septations, and they are removed to minimize the risk of future sinus disease. This should be performed with a diamond burr to protect the dura if invaginations are present. Ensure that no portion of the sinus is left without a drainage tract. The anterior table itself may need to be contoured as its thickness allows when the superciliary arches are prominent. After contouring, the anterior table segment is replaced in a more recessed position. The technique chosen for osteosynthesis is based on surgeon preference. The author currently use 0.6 mm titanium midface plates with monocortical screws of the minimum length needed. The plating pattern will vary based on the fit of the free bone segment with 1 to 3 small linear plates used in most cases. Resorbable plating systems are a viable option, though the plates are often palpable and occasionally visible for several months. When the free anterior table segment is replaced, it is unlikely to be perfectly flush with the frontal bone around its entire perimeter, but any small gaps should be minimized to the extent possible. Shavings from the bone contouring are collected and used to fill any residual interspace between the bones.

As the desired outcome is to create not just plausibly feminine facial proportions, but undeniably feminine ones, a setback of the anterior table of the frontal sinus is required in nearly all patients. In a minority of patients that present with minimal anterior projection of the brow bone, a type I reduction with contouring alone may achieve the desired result. Type II reductions with bone cement applied to the mid-forehead are rarely performed as additional bone contouring can typically create the desired round forehead shape without the risk of an implant. Type IV procedures are also rare. If performed, methyl methacrylate is no longer the best material available for augmentation. The author has never found it necessary to use either type II or type IV procedures, but has used autologous fat grafting to augment and round the central forehead to subtly improve upper facial proportions in patients who had a previous surgical reduction.

CREATING A MORE FEMININE EYEBROW POSITION

The shape and location of the ideal feminine eyebrow will be discussed in greater depth elsewhere in this issue, but it is higher and with a more elevated tail than a masculine eyebrow position. The process of lowering the hairline by excising a strip of tissue from the inferior flap will elevate the eyebrows. It is rare, though, that the tissue excision needed to create the ideal hairline shape is the same as that needed to create the ideal eyebrow symmetry, shape, and position. In fact, preoperatively, the higher eyebrow is most often on the side with the higher hairline. There are several techniques that can be used to uncouple the movement of these 2 structures. The hair bearing flap can be undermined asymmetrically, so that the side with higher hairline is more mobile. Scoring of the galea for the superior flap, or the periosteum of the lower flap can also independently mobilize a region. Monocortical bone tunnels, bioabsorbable anchors, or other fixation devices can be used to limit or augment the movement of either flap. Brow height should be over corrected, as there is always some postoperative descent.

DISCUSSION
Is Preoperative Imaging Required?

There is some disagreement about the role of preoperative imaging for GCFS. Surgeons who routinely order imaging will point out that it can be a valuable aid when

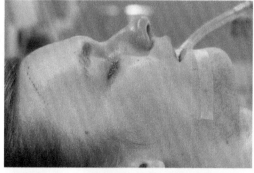

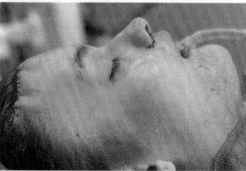

Fig. 1. Immediate intraoperative result.

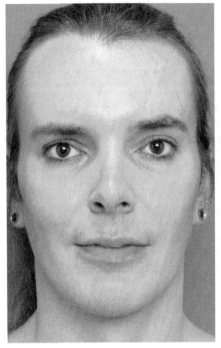
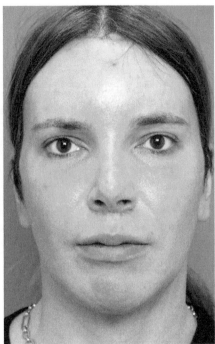

Fig. 2. 1 month after surgery frontal.

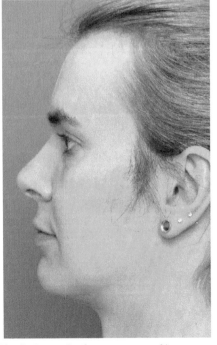
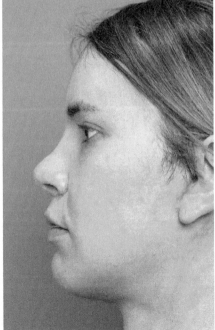

Fig. 3. 1 month after surgery profile.

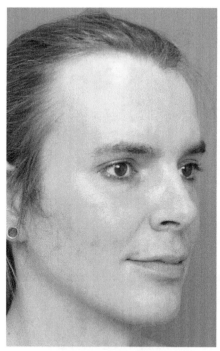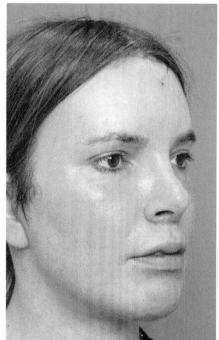

Fig. 4. 1 month after surgery 45.

used in the preoperative consultation. Preoperative knowledge of the frontal sinus dimensions and confirming the absence of abnormal dural invaginations could potentially decrease operative time. There are even several jig or cutting guide systems offered that are custom fabricated and require CT imaging. Surgeons that do not routinely order imaging argue that the benefits are not worth the costs. Proper technique should allow the surgeon to enter the sinus in the proper location without imaging. With cautious bone removal, abnormalities such as dural invaginations or venous lakes should be evident before they are disrupted. The author is in the latter group. Currently GCFS is not well covered by health insurance in the US. Hence, patients face an unpredictable out of pocket expese. That cost, in addition to the radiation dose associated with the procedure, does not seem to justify the minimal benefits. As insurance coverage improves and radiation doses continue to decrease, it may better balance that equation at some point in the future. When referring a patient for GCFS, I would not recommend ordering imaging unless familiar with that surgeon's preferences.

Is Hair Grafting or Hairline Advancement the Best Option?

A hairline advancement allows the surgeon to bring full-length hair into a more feminine shape and location. A surgical hairline advancement is included in 95% of forehead feminization procedures performed in the autor's practice. The hairline scar heals well in most patients, but hairline scar revision is also the most common revision surgery after GCFS in this practice. Hair grafting can produce the same hairline changes, but typically with a longer timeframe and higher cost. If a patient is going to have hair grafting performed, it is best conducted after GCFS in most patients. Scarring from transplant harvest and placement can complicate tissue elevation

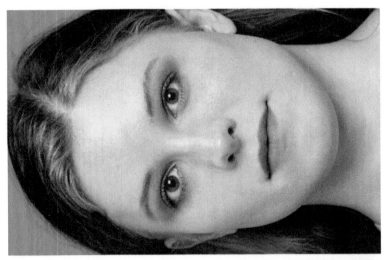

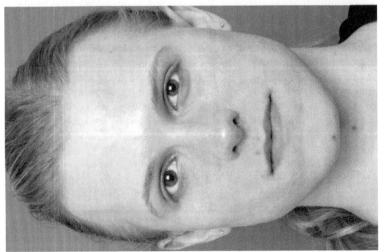

Fig. 5. 3 months after surgery frontal.

and limit mobility. If a patient is interested in changing their hairline in addition to the contour of their forehead, they should understand both options, but it is recommended they consult with their GCF surgeon before a hair transplant is performed.

What "Type" of Forehead Reduction is Needed?

The anterior table of the frontal sinus is typically only 2 to 3 mm thick at its thinnest point. When it is thicker, any modification should leave most or the anterior at least 2 to 3 mm thick so that it is not overly prone to fracture. A type 1 reduction, or just "shaving" the brow bone, can only result in minimal contour change unless the frontal sinus is hypoplastic with an unusually thick anterior table. A type 3 reduction with a setback of the anterior table is almost always required to correct any significant brow bossing with a typical anterior table thickness. One argument for preoperative imaging is that it allows the surgeon to confirm what type of forehead reduction will be performed. If past imaging has not been performed patients are advised that they will most likely require a type 3 reduction, but a setback will be avoided if the desired contour can be achieved while still leaving adequate anterior table thickness. The recovery and postsurgical risks of type 1 and type 3 reductions are not significantly different.

What are the Risks of Brow Bone Reduction?

Regardless of the location of the access incision or type of bone reduction performed, brow bone reduction is a safe outpatient procedure with a very low risk of acute complications. Hematoma is a hypothetical risk, though elevation in the avascular subperiosteal plane minimizes this. A violation of the dura while contouring or placing bone anchors is rare and should be recognized intraoperatively. Beyond acute issues,

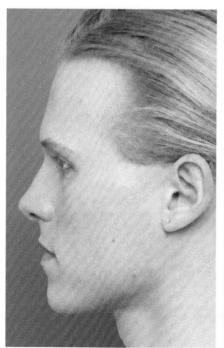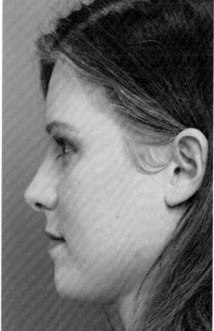

Fig. 6. 3 months after surgery profile.

hairline scar widening is the most common complication seen. In the author's practice, revision of this scar is the most common reason for surgical revision after GCFS in general. While the patient numbers and length of follow up seen in GCFS studies are often not what is seen in studies in other fields, chronic frontal sinus complications are quite rare (**Figs. 1–6** Video 1).[10,11]

SUMMARY

The reduction of brow bossing is a powerful GCFS. Most patients will need a type 3 reduction with a setback of the anterior table of the frontal sinus to get the best result possible. Brow bone reduction is always paired with the reduction of the orbital rims and is often paired with adjustments to the hairline and eyebrow position. The procedure is a safe outpatient surgery with few acute or chronic complications.

PEARLS

- The reduction of a prominent brow ridge will make a face more likely to be perceived as feminine than any other change in facial structure.
- Forehead feminization typically includes the reduction of the brow ridge along with the adjustment of the hairline and eyebrows.
- Most patients will require a setback of the frontal table of the anterior sinus to achieve an optimal outcome.
- Brow reduction is a safe surgical procedure that is not associated with major short- or long-term complications.

DISCLOSURE

The authors have nothing to disclose.

SUPPLEMENTARY DATA

Supplementary data related to this article can be found online at https://doi.org/10.1016/j.otc.2022.04.003.

REFERENCES

1. Spiegel JH. Facial determinants of female gender and feminizing forehead cranioplasty. Laryngoscope 2011;121:250–61.
2. Ousterhout DK. Feminization of the forehead: contour changing to improve female aesthetics. Plast Reconstr Surg 1987;79(5):701–13.
3. Rodman R, Sturm AK. Hairline restoration: difference in men and woman-length and shape. Facial Plast Surg 2018;34(2):155–8.
4. Lee MK, Sakai O, Spiegel JH. CT measurement of the frontal sinus - gender differences and implications for frontal cranioplasty. J Craniomaxillofac Surg 2010;38:494–500.
5. Capitán L, Simon D, Kaye K, et al. Facial feminization surgery: the forehead. Surgical techniques and analysis of results. Plast Reconstr Surg 2014;134(4):609–19.
6. Capitan L, Simon D, Meyer T, et al. Facial feminization surgery: simultaneous hair transplant during forehead reconstruction. Plast Reconstr Surg 2017;139:573–84.

7. Garcia-Rodriguez L, Thain LM, Spiegel JH. Scalp advancement for transgender women: closing the gap. Laryngoscope 2019;130:1431–5.

8. Jung S, Oh SJ, Hoon Koh S. Hair follicle transplantation on scar tissue. J Craniofac Surg 2013;24(4):1239–41.

9. Kleinberger AJ, Jumaily J, Spiegel JH. Safety of modified coronal approach with dissection deep to temporalis fascia for facial nerve preservation. Otolaryngol Head Neck Surg 2015;152(4):655–60.

10. Basa K, Lee A, Shehan JN, et al. Frontal bone cranioplasty for facial feminization: long-term follow-up of postoperative sinonasal symptoms. Facial Plast Surg Aesthet Med 2021. https://doi.org/10.1089/fpsam.2021.0037.

11. Eggerstedt M, Hong YS, Wakefield CJ, et al. Setbacks in forehead feminization cranioplasty: a systematic review of complications and patient-reported outcomes. Aesthetic Plast Surg 2020;44(3):743–9.

Brow Lift and Brow Position for Gender Affirmation

Michael Somenek, MD*, Nahir J. Romero, MD

KEYWORDS

- Brow lift • Brow positioning • Female/male brow
- Brow positioning gender affirmation

KEY POINTS

- It is important to recognize the characteristic differences between male and female eyebrows to achieve desirable results during gender affirmation interventions.
- Knowledge of facial anatomy is a key to recognize the levels and planes of dissection for each particular approach.
- Know pros and cons of different approaches to pair these with patients' expectations and obtain the best outcomes.

INTRODUCTION

If the eyes are considered by some as the windows to the soul, the eyebrows can then be the frames that adorn them and can help accentuate a person's facial features. They are a staple of attractiveness, conveying emotion and projecting personality traits. Therefore, the utmost attention and intimate understanding of their role is required when modifying them to achieve an esthetically pleasing result. When discussing gender affirmation surgery, the eyebrows play a key role. As a key gender-associated recognizable feature, they add to the balance and contour of an individual's face. Great care should be taken not to alter their functionality when attempting a cosmetic modification.

When the face is divided into thirds, the upper third extends from the glabella to the trichion (**Fig. 1**). The youthful brow region must be full and convex with soft skin and no rhytids. On a three-quarter view, the convex brow transitions softly into a concave lateral orbital wall and forms the upper facial ogee. On a frontal view, the temple is full and prevents visualization of the zygomatic arch or temporal line. The brow fat span (BFS) and the tarsal platform show (TPS) represent the distance between the upper eyebrow and upper lid crease as well as the lid crease and upper eyelid margin, respectively. A youthful appearing individual has a TPS:BFS ratio of 1:1.5 medially and 1:3 laterally.[1]

Advanced Plastic Surgery, 2440 M Street Northwest, Suite 507, Washington, DC 20037, USA
* Corresponding author.
E-mail address: drsomenek@spmeddc.com

Otolaryngol Clin N Am 55 (2022) 797–808
https://doi.org/10.1016/j.otc.2022.04.004
0030-6665/22/© 2022 Elsevier Inc. All rights reserved.

oto.theclinics.com

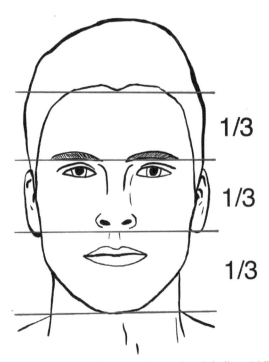

1/3

1/3

1/3

Fig. 1. Facial thirds. Upper third goes from trichion to the glabella, middle third goes from the glabella to subnasale, and lower third goes from subnasale to menton.

BACKGROUND: FACIAL ANALYSIS

When planning for gender affirmation surgery, some important differences regarding facial analysis should be taken into account in order to obtain the most desirable results. In general, the female skull is smaller and rounder than the male skull.[2,3] Dividing the face into thirds and following a top-to-bottom analysis can be a valuable method for developing a surgical plan.[4] For the purpose of this article, we focus on the analysis of the upper third of the face. Areas of importance in this region include the hairline, forehead, and the brow region.

When evaluating the hairline, the shape as well as the length of it is important. Feminine hairlines tend to be fuller and have a smoother contour. There is a shorter distance between the nasion and hairline of approximately 1 cm (averaging 5 cm for females, 6 cm for males).[5] Male hairlines can be receding, have a widow's peak or M-shape configuration.[6]

When analyzing the forehead, the surgeon must take into account its length, bossing, convexity, and nasofrontal angle. With regards to the female esthetic, the forehead tends to have a smooth and softer convexity. In contrast, males will commonly exhibit supraorbital bossing and a broader, more prominent convexity. The medial supraorbital ridge blends into the glabella resulting in greater projection and an overall more masculine appearance.[7,8] The naso-glabellar region represents the transition between forehead and nose. This area needs to be taken into account as it is a key component in bringing harmony and balance between the upper and middle thirds of the face.[9] In males, their nasofrontal angle is more acute, creating a sharper transition in this region of the face. Females tend to possess a smoother convexity from orbit to vertex, with minimal supraorbital bossing and a nasofrontal angle that is more obtuse.[7,10]

When it comes to brow position, the female brow possesses a few distinctive characteristics. The medial limit is located at or below the orbital rim, with a straight medial brow segment. It begins at a line drawn from the alar crease through the medial canthus. The brow then begins to peak at a takeoff angle of 15° to 25°. The brow peak is located at the lateral canthus for younger women whereas, in an older patient, the brow peak can be more medial.[3,4,9] The eyebrow also sits higher in a female patient, slightly above the supraorbital rim. In the previous decades, it was desirable for the zenith, highest point or the eyebrow, to be located more medially (above the lateral limbus). The lateral portion usually lays 1 to 2 mm above the medial aspect.[11]

In males, the eyebrow lies at the level of the supraorbital rim and is less arched. When contrasted to the female brow, they are typically more inferior in position, having a fuller or thicker hair content and overall flatter appearance. The supraorbital ridge is generally more pronounced in masculine faces with a less steep slant from the supraorbital ridge to the vertex[6,12,13] **(Fig. 2)**.

DISCUSSION

Approaches to brow shaping have changed significantly over the past several decades. More recent advances have allowed for a decrease in visible scars, complications, and healing time.[14,15] The proper selection and best option regarding the approach will depend on the patient's personalized appearance and needs. Functional and cosmetic concerns should also be taken into account.

During the preoperative evaluation for an eyebrow procedure, it is always important to inquire about prior treatments to the area. A history of previous neurotoxin to the frontalis or upper face within the last 6 months is especially important as this can alter the baseline relationship of the scalp, brow, and eyelid position.

Different Approaches

When discussing different approaches to brow surgery, it is helpful to understand that the surgeon will have better control over the final brow position the closer the incision site is to the brow. The chosen technique must be weighed against variables such as patient expectations, visibility of the scar, and risk of complications **(Fig. 3)**.

For all different techniques, important operative risks and pitfalls should be recognized and avoided. The most important objective is always to find the correct plane of dissection. The surgeon will need to understand exactly which surgical plane is necessary to achieve the desired results. Each brow lift technique requires unique and often multiple levels of dissection.

Depending on the approach selected, careful anatomic dissection and conservative use of cautery and traction should be performed in the region of the frontal branch of the facial nerve path to preserve it. The frontal branch of the facial nerve travels just deep to the temporoparietal fascia above the zygomatic arch and advances up and lateral on its trajectory to innervate the frontalis muscle. Anatomic studies suggest that the nerve branch becomes more superficial approximately 1.5 cm above the arch and 1 cm from the lateral orbital rim.[16] This location will put it at risk during brow lift procedures. The nerve will be best protected by the surgeon elevating on the plane right on the temporalis fascia. This way the nerve will be safely elevated and protected with the temporoparietal fascia. This is warranted to help avoid injury and resulting paralysis to this region of the face **(Fig. 4)**.

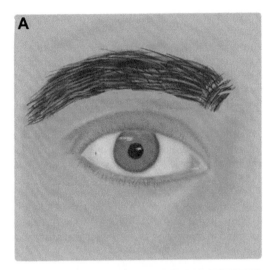

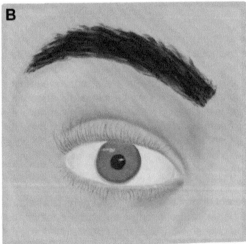

Fig. 2. Male vs female eyebrow placement. (*A*) In males, the eyebrow lies at the level of the supraorbital rim and is less arched. They have a thicker hair content and overall flatter appearance. (*B*) In females, the medial limit is located at or below the orbital rim. The brow peak is located at the lateral canthus for younger women whereas in the older patient it can be more medially. The eyebrow also sits higher in a younger woman, slightly above the supraorbital rim.

For all the approaches, it is useful to mark the incision sites with the patient in an upright position. The chosen anesthetic is 1% lidocaine with 1:100,000 epinephrine and the author's preference for sterile prep is half-strength betadine solution.

Direct brow lift
This approach will be a good choice for patients that may not be as concerned with scars. Older patients with significant brow ptosis or thick and abundant eyebrow hair are great candidates for this approach. They will have the advantage of better scar camouflage as their thick hair can immediately conceal the incision resulting

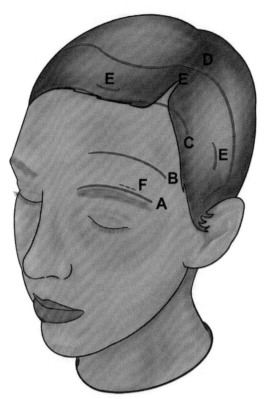

Fig. 3. Approaches: (A) direct brow lift, (B) midforehead, (C) hairline brow lift or pretrichial, (D) coronal brow lift, (E) endoscopic brow lift, and (F) browpexy.

from this approach. Another benefit of this approach is that it will grant the greatest control of lift to the entire brow complex, especially the angulation laterally. It also preserves forehead sensation. However, this approach may not be the best option to perform simultaneously with other facial feminization procedures. If the patient will be undergoing forehead or orbital rim remodeling to feminize the facial bony framework, it will not be desirable to have osteotomies and bony modifications immediately under an open-healing incision.

A horizontal incision is created following the eyebrow shape along and inside the upper row of hairs in the brow hairline. Care should be taken to bevel the incision in the direction of the hair shafts to prevent hair loss near the incision. This will also help create an everted skin closure. The length of the incision should not extend past the superior brow hair-bearing margin. Superior edge subcutaneous dissection can be completed to improve forehead rhytids in this region if needed. Detachment of the affected skin from the deeper forehead muscle activity will allow improvement in static rhytids. After hemostasis is achieved with bipolar cautery, the orbicularis and frontalis muscles may be plicated and sutured to the periosteum of the lower forehead using multiple well-positioned 4 to 0 Polydioxanone Suture (PDS) simple sutures to achieve adequate correction of brow ptosis along lateral, central, and medial aspects. The excess skin is removed and the dermal closure is then performed using 5 to 0 PDS simple subcutaneous sutures oriented to create eversion of the wound edges. The skin is closed with 6 to 0 Prolene in a simple interrupted fashion.

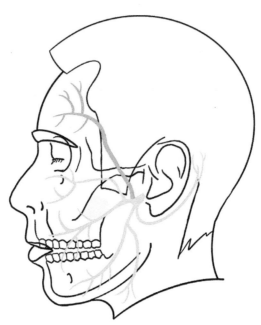

Fig. 4. Frontal branch of the facial nerve. It travels just deep to the temporoparietal fascia above the zygomatic arch and advances up and lateral on its trajectory to innervate the frontalis muscle. Anatomic studies suggest the nerve branch becomes more superficial approximately 1.5 cm above the arch and 1 cm from the lateral orbital rim.

The downside to using this technique is a potentially visible scar. However, meticulous closure along the beveled incision can help minimize scar formations.

Midforehead

This approach is good for unpredictable hairlines and patients with preexisting forehead rhytids. The presence of deeper rhytids will help to camouflage the resulting scar. Incision placement allows wide access to the forehead tissues inferiorly that can be easily freed above the brow complex. This approach grants an excellent control of positioning along the entire brow. It is considered to be somewhat better than direct brow lift at addressing medial brow/glabellar ptosis. It is also good for patients with receding or unpredictable hairlines as this area will be preserved by using the midforehead approach. Even though the approach will grant exposure to the forehead and supraorbital ridge, it may not be the best option to perform simultaneously with other facial feminization procedures. Like previously mentioned with the direct approach, if the patient will be undergoing forehead or orbital rim remodeling to feminize the facial bony framework, it will not be desirable to have osteotomies and bony modifications immediately under an open-healing incision.

A crescent horizontal incision is created in the midforehead taking care to bevel the incision to allow for eversion of the skin. The contralateral incision should be planned in an asymmetric fashion, choosing an alternative rhytid height, which will allow for greater camouflage (**Fig. 5**). The horizontal length of the incision can be extended medially, with some overlap if needed, to correct severe medial forehead/glabellar ptosis.[17]

Limited subcutaneous superior dissection will allow some eversion of the skin margin. The inferior subcutaneous undermining may be carried more extensively if

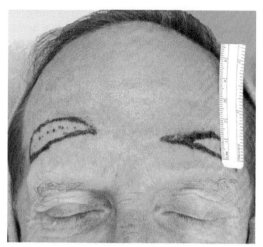

Fig. 5. Midforehead lift incision planning, placement, and orientation.

necessary. Great care must be taken with medial dissection to avoid the supraorbital neurovascular bundle as well as with lateral dissection to avoid injury to the frontal branch of the facial nerve. The amount of skin removed will be based on the lift required. Fixation is achieved using a 4 to 0 PDS to secure the orbicularis to the superior periosteum as well as the soft tissues of the brow. The skin closure is performed with the same technique as the direct brow lift.

The downside to using this technique is a potentially visible scar. However, meticulous closure and adjunctive therapies such as microneedling can help to maximize the appearance of the scar, making it quite imperceptible within the natural architecture of the forehead rhytids.

Hairline brow lift (pretrichial)
The pretrichial brow lift is a great option for patients with a prominent forehead who would benefit from a hairline advancement as this technique lowers the hairline position. The excess skin will be removed anterior to the hairline incision resulting in a forward advancement of the previous hairline location. This makes a patient with a high hairline a good candidate. Another advantage of the technique is that it allows for excellent elevation of the full brow to correct lateral orbital hooding, glabellar skin ptosis, and corrugator- and procerus-induced rhytids.[3] It can also help correct disproportions of the upper third of the face. This technique can be very useful for a patient who will be undergoing other simultaneous facial feminization procedures in the upper third of the face and can be perform at the same time. It will provide a good exposure for bony framework modifications, and at the same time, modifications and advancement of the hairlaine can be performed if the patient needs them.

The hairline incision should be carefully planned in advance. It should be designed in an irregularly undulating or broken geometric pattern so that results are optimal and most natural-looking. This will be similar to the incisions designed for hairline advancement or hair transplant. The incision is created a few millimeters behind the hairline in a beveled fashion. Cutting across the anterior hair follicles will allow hair to grow through the skin closure to aid in concealing the scar. The exposure and dissection are facilitated anteriorly and inferiorly in the subgaleal plane up to 3 cm above the brow. The dissection plane then changes to the subperiosteal plane and continues down to the nasal bones. Care must be taken to preserve the supraorbital and supratrochlear neurovascular bundles. The lateral incision extends to the temple hair. In this area, dissection is carried down to the superficial layer of the deep temporal fascia. Anterior dissection to the orbital rim is carried out under the temporoparietal fascia where the frontal branch of the facial nerve is contained.[18] The arcus marginalis is released at the level of the orbital rim, which permits mobilization of the lateral brow. An adequate amount of skin is excised anterior to the incision.

A disadvantage of this technique is it may result in a more visible scar. However, as previously discussed, meticulous closure and adjunctive therapies can help make the scar less noticeable.

Coronal brow lift

The coronal brow lift can be very useful for a patient who will be undergoing other simultaneous facial feminization procedures in the upper third of the face, as this is the preferred approach that is used for forehead contouring. The coronal incision, as well as the previously discussed pretrichial approach, allows for an excellent elevation of the full brow, and exposure to the bony structures of the forehead and orbital ridge are the most desirable ones. It can correct a variety of abnormalities including lateral orbital hooding, glabellar skin ptosis, and corrugator- and procerus-induced rhytids.

The curvilinear coronal incision is placed in a position such that it will be located roughly 3 cm posterior to the hairline after the removal of 1 to 2 cm of skin anteriorly. The incision should be created parallel to the hair follicles. The lateral extension of the incision may extend to the level of the helical root. The rest of the technique will be the same as previously discussed for the pretrichial approach. Some surgeons recommend using tissue adhesives or bone-anchoring techniques for additional brow support during the healing phase.[19] Some studies have revealed fixation with sutures produces more stable results than glue without greater risks.[20]

A potential disadvantage of this technique is it will raise the position of the hairline and increase the vertical length of the upper third of the face. These should be taken into consideration during the patient selection. It also has a higher risk of permanent hypoesthesia of the scalp.

Endoscopic brow lift

The endoscopic brow lift technique allows for reduced, well-camouflaged incisions behind the temporal and frontal hairlines. This makes it an excellent option for younger patients without prominent rhytids and others that desire maximum scar camouflage. It will also preserve the hairline and provide access to all different aspects of the eyebrow. In addition, it reduces the risk of potential forehead and scalp numbness. The approach provides central and lateral oblique vectors, which grant the capacity to exert multi-vector lift forces and brow correction.[16] This approach may also permit for earlier resolution of tissue swelling and less blood loss.[14] This approach will be hard to combine with other upper facial feminization procedures because the exposure for bony remodeling using these small incisions and the scope will be very limited.

Two weeks before the procedure, the neurotoxin is administered to the brow depressors (glabella, lateral orbicularis, and frontalis muscles). This will decrease the inferior pull on the forehead tissues and relax the forehead complex, whereas the periosteum is healing in the elevated position.

Dissection is facilitated medially using a central horizontal incision (1.5 cm) and two vertical incisions (2 cm) over the intended apex of the lateral brow.[14] Direct subperiosteal dissection is carried using a curved periosteal elevator down to a level approximately 1.5 cm above the orbital rims. Dissection is carried posteriorly toward the vertex of the scalp. Temporal incisions are obliquely fashioned for lateral dissection. The appropriate dissection plane will be on the surface of the superficial layer of the deep temporal fascia overlying the temporalis muscle. This permits wide field elevation of the flap to a point lateral to the orbital rim (roughly 2 cm). Using a 30° endoscope, division of the conjoint tendon between the medial subperiosteal and lateral subgaleal planes at the superior temporal line is performed. To allow superior mobilization of the brows, the forehead tissue must be released from the bone and deep fascia. The confluence of fascia along the conjoint tendon makes dissection more difficult laterally. When dissecting toward the lateral canthus during the anterior dissection, care should be taken to preserve the sentinel vein. Not preserving it could predispose the patient to more noticeable and visible superficial periorbital/temple veins postoperatively. A branch of the temporozygomatic sensory nerve often accompanies this vein as well. Damage may cause needless numbness in the zygomatic area. To maintain long-term results using this technique, the precanthal ligament and superior orbital ligament must be released. The release of periosteum at the level of the orbital rim, glabella, and the superior temporal crest is facilitated endoscopically. Great care must be taken to spare the supraorbital neurovascular structures. The corrugator, procerus, and depressor supercilii can be divided simultaneously. Care must be taken to not over resect the corrugator muscle. This can lead to an unpleasing widened interbrow distance. Some surgeons advise in favor of completing a horizontal myotomy of the orbicularis oculi. This will not only weaken the orbicularis oculi muscle and its pull on the eyebrow but also interrupt the innervation to the corrugator supercilii muscle and prevent its downward pull on the eyebrow as well.[15,21]

Lateral fixation is achieved using a 3 to 0 PDS to secure the anterior temporal flap to the temporalis fascia in an oblique vector postero-superiorly. Central fixation can be achieved in the two paramedian vertical incisions using a couple of options. The endotine fixation system is an easy-to-use bone anchor that absorbs over time. It provides the temporary superior fixation to the brow, forehead, and scalp tissues. Alternatively, a cortical tunnel system can be used which allows suture fixation of forehead skin to a channel drilled into the outer cortex of the skull. Incisions are closed superficially with a resorbable suture.

When evaluating for patient selection, patients with a convex forehead may prove not to be the best candidates for this approach. The main reason is that the endoscope may not be able to visualize the inferior medial anatomy. It is also not ideal for patients with a high hairline position because it may be elevated further and a relatively high point of fixation may limit control of the brow shape. A potential disadvantage of this technique is that the use of the endotine fixation system and preoperative neurotoxin may add expenses to this approach.

Browpexy

This approach seeks to elevate or stabilize the brow via a direct and minimally invasive approach. This approach will work great for a patient that is looking to get the most minimally invasive approach but still see some controlled lift. This approach is particularly beneficial for patients looking to raise the lateral brow for a feminizing effect. Patients with thick and abundant eyebrow hair will conceal the small incision very well. This technique offers a minimally invasive approach providing rapid recovery and long-lasting elevation of the brow.[22,23]

It will be a good option for patients looking for a feminizing effect to the eyebrow, but not extensive work or modifications to the bony frame as the incision and exposure with this approach are meant to be minimal.

Internal browpexy was first described as a brow suspension performed in conjunction with upper blepharoplasty through the same incision.[21] Zandi and colleagues demonstrated effective, long-lasting elevation comparable or better than temporal brow lifts in female patients[23.] The brow fat and orbicularis muscle are raised and secured to the periosteum more superiorly.

External browpexy relies on an 8-mm incision along the central superior edge of the eyebrow. Through this small cutaneous access, a 2.5-cm wide transverse cut is made through the orbicularis muscle and brow fat down to the periosteum.[24,25] A 4 to 0 permanent horizontal mattress suture is passed through the periosteum at the desired brow height. The suture is then passed through the orbicularis and brow fat at the inferior extent of the dissection. The suture is tied, and the incision is closed in two layers. After external browpexy, the brow should resist inferior displacement. Transpalpebral browpexy involves the resection of the lateral orbicularis oculi and release of the lateral brow-retaining ligaments. This will make the frontalis unopposed like it was previously discussed with the endoscopic technique, providing great results.

Potential disadvantages of this technique can be prolonged eyelid edema and possible brow asymmetry.

CLINICS CARE POINTS

- Asymmetry of brow position: This should be identified and corrected if possible, during the initial evaluation. Many preoperative asymmetries are noted to be functional. They can be an unconscious imbalanced activity from the frontalis muscle.

- Injury to the frontal branch of the facial nerve: This can result in significant, dramatic, and disfiguring upper facial asymmetry. Great care should be taken in the elevation of tissues and understanding the proper anatomic planes as previously discussed when dissecting close to the trajectory of the facial nerve.

- Paresthesia or numbness of the forehead: Direct, midforehead, and hairline incision approaches may result in numbness above the level of the incision. During manipulation of the neurovascular bundle using the endoscopic, coronal, or trichophytic approach, great care should be taken to preserve these structures. Tension or pull on the nerve often leads to some supraorbital or supratrochlear neural dysfunction. The sensation may return even up to a year out from the procedure.

- Hair loss: Incisions created behind the hairline are usually well concealed and heal well. Hair loss around incision sites is possible, especially with overuse of cautery around the hair follicles. Gentle tissue handling techniques and minimization of cautery use will help avoid this issue.

ACKNOWLEDGMENTS

Illustrators: Andy J. Martinez, MD, Natalie May, MS.

DISCLOSURE

No disclosures.

REFERENCES

1. Flint PW, Cummings CW, Nassif P. Cummings otolaryngology: head and neck surgery: the aesthetic brow and forehead. Philadelphia, PA: Elsevier; 2021. p. 388–401.
2. Rafaty FM, Brennan HG. Current concepts of browpexy. Arch Otolaryngol 1983; 109:152.
3. Van den Bosch WA, Leenders I, Mulder P. Topographic anatomy of the eyelids, and the effects of sex and age. Br J Ophthalmol 1999;83:347–52.
4. Matros E, Garcia JA, Yaremchuk MJ. Changes in eyebrow position and shape with aging. Plast Reconstr Surg 2009;124(4):1296–301.
5. Scheuer JF 3rd, Matarasso A, Rohrich RJ. Optimizing male periorbital rejuvenation. Dermatol Surg 2017;43(Suppl 2):S196–202.
6. Lakhiani C, Somenek MT. Gender-related facial analysis. Facial Plast Surg Clin North Am 2019;27(2):171–7.
7. Ousterhout DK. Feminization of the forehead: contour changing to improve female aesthetics. Plast Reconstr Surg 1987;79(5):701–13.
8. Hage JJ, Becking AG, de Graaf FH, et al. Gender-confirming facial surgery: considerations on the masculinity and femininity of faces. Plast Reconstr Surg 1997; 99(7):1799–807.
9. Capitán L, Simon D, Kaye K, et al. Facial feminization surgery: the forehead. Surgical techniques and analysis of results. Plast Reconstr Surg 2014;134(4): 609–19.
10. Dempf R, Eckert AW. Contouring the forehead and rhinoplasty in the feminization of the face in male-to-female transsexuals. J Craniomaxillofac Surg 2010;38(6): 416–22.
11. Sedgh J. The aesthetics of the upper face and brow: male and female differences. Facial Plast Surg 2018;34(2):114–8.
12. Cho SW, Jin HR. Feminization of the forehead in a transgender: frontal sinus reshaping combined with brow lift and hairline lowering. Aesthetic Plast Surg 2012; 36(5):1207–10.
13. Becking AG, Tuinzing DB, Hage JJ, et al. Transgender feminization of the facial skeleton. Clin Plast Surg 2007;34(3):557–64.
14. Isse N. Endoscopic facial rejuvenation: endoforehead the functional lift-brief update. Aesthetic Plast Surg 2020;44(4):1171–2.
15. De la Fuente A, Santamaría AB. Endoscopic forehead lift: is it effective? Aesthet Surg J 2002;22(2):113–20.
16. Myers Eugene N, Ricardo L. Carrau. *operative otolaryngology: head and neck surgery. Brow lift* Philadelphia: Saunders/Elsevier; 2008.
17. Cook TA, Brownrigg PJ, Wang TD, et al. The versatile midforehead browlift. Arch Otolaryngol Head Neck Surg 1989;115(2):163–8.
18. Adamson PA, Johnson CM Jr, Anderson JR, et al. The forehead lift. a review. Arch Otolaryngol 1985;111(5):325–9.
19. Stuzin JM, Wagstrom L, Kawamoto HK, et al. Anatomy of the frontal branch of the facial nerve: the significance of the temporal fat pad. Plast Reconstr Surg 1989; 83(2):265–71.
20. Jones BM, Grover R. Endoscopic brow lift: a personal review of 538 patients and comparison of fixation techniques. Plast Reconstr Surg 2004;113(4):1242–52.
21. Perkins SW, Batniji RK. Trichophytic endoscopic forehead-lifting in high hairline patients. Facial Plast Surg Clin North Am 2006;14(3):185–93.

22. McCord CD, Doxanas MT. Browplasty and browpexy: an adjunct to blepharo-plasty. Plast Reconstr Surg 1990;86(2):248–54.
23. Zandi A, Ranjbar-Omidi B, Pourazizi M. Temporal brow lift vs internal browpexy in females undergoing upper blepharoplasty: Effects on lateral brow lifting. J Cosmet Dermatol 2018;17(5):855–61.
24. Massry GG. The external browpexy. Ophthalmic Plast Reconstr Surg 2012;28(2):90–5.
25. Ogilvie MP, Few JW Jr, Semersky AJ, et al. What neurotoxins have taught us about the brow: the reintroduction and review of the transpalpebral browpexy. Aesthetic Plast Surg 2018;42(1):126–36.

Feminization Rhinoplasty

Jesús Báez-Márquez, MD

KEYWORDS

- Rhinoplasty • Feminization rhinoplasty • Transgender • Facial feminization surgery
- Gender confirmation surgery • Gender-affirming surgery

KEY POINTS

- Author's approach to transgender rhinoplasty.
- Patients seek the most natural and functional results with feminization rhinoplasty.
- Combining rhinoplasty with frontal bone remodeling achieves the most optimal results for transgender women.
- Preservation of nasal ligaments, hemi-transdomal sutures, resting angle concept, and anterior nasal septal angle grafts achieves long-lasting and natural results.

INTRODUCTION

Facial gender affirmation surgery is currently growing worldwide and is an important treatment for gender dysphoria that will improve quality of life.[1] The most frequently sought modifications by transgender women are forehead and supraorbital ridge reduction, cheek augmentation, upper lip surgery (lip lift), laryngeal chondroplasty, jaw reduction, and rhinoplasty.[2]

Rhinoplasty for transgender women uses the same techniques as rhinoplasty for a cisgender patient. However, knowledge of transgender care is necessary and must be widely adapted to all health professionals.[3] This article intends to explain the author's personal approach to feminization rhinoplasty.

PREOPERATIVE PLANNING
Consultation

It's very important to educate patients about the procedures that may be needed to reach their goals. Nevertheless, all surgeries must be personalized, and the surgeon must understand the patient's needs and desires, and, as surgeons, we must give treatment options. Rhinoplasty as a procedure for facial feminization is not enough. For transgender women, it is suggested to operate glabellar/orbital rim reduction and rhinoplasty during the same surgical time, because in this way we achieve a more balanced and feminine nasofrontal angle.

Avenida Empresarios 150, Interior 2305, Puerta de Hierro, Zapopan, Jalisco, CP 45116, Mexico
E-mail address: drjesus@facecenter.mx

Otolaryngol Clin N Am 55 (2022) 809–823
https://doi.org/10.1016/j.otc.2022.04.005
0030-6665/22/© 2022 Elsevier Inc. All rights reserved.

oto.theclinics.com

Although some patients may search for drastic transformation, the majority of transgender women are looking for the most natural, non-noticeable technique. They desire to be free of any kind of surgical stigma for best passing.

For achieving a feminine facial appearance in both cis and transgender patients, the forehead ideally must have a smooth continuous curvature and more obtuse nasofrontal angle. It's essential to address any supraorbital bossing that doesn't match a feminine appearance and bring balance to the profile.[4] Just after forehead and orbital remodeling, proceed to rhinoplasty, although there is no problem with performing rhinoplasty at a second operative time afterward.

Patients treated with hormone replacement therapy for at least 1 year may experience an improvement in skin softening, less facial hair growth, reduced production of sebum, and thinning of the skin;[5] therefore, the results of rhinoplasty will be more satisfactory overall. Although 1 year of hormone therapy is a goal for all patients, it is not a requirement.

Routine preoperative assessment of a patient undergoing facial feminization surgery (FFS), as well as postoperative imaging assessment if needed, involves a computed tomography (CT) of the facial bones without contrast, which provides greater anatomic detail and improved three-dimesional characterization of the face than X-ray.[6] A preoperative CT scan is essential to determine the shape and size of the frontal sinus and its relation to the orbita, nasal bones, nasal septum, and posterior wall of the frontal sinus. This is especially helpful if the patient has had a previous frontal bone remodeling procedure, assessing for any weakness near the frontal osteoplastic flap and searching intentionally for any skull base sequelae of the previous surgery.

A complete physical exam of the face and photo documentation are done at the pre-op visit. The photo is studied alongside the patient as they voice their concerns. This is the time to notify the patient of what can and what cannot be done. Never elevate a patient's expectations, just be concise and honest.

Preoperative computer simulation rhinoplasty software is a common tool nowadays. The simulation must be intended for surgical planning, analysis, and communication with patients.[7] The simulated result must be a conservative idea, not a perfect result and should represent near accuracy to the surgeons' real cases and not mimic third-party results. If during the simulation the patient requests unrealistic results, doesn't like the surgeons simulation, asks for too many changes or even "leads" the simulation, these could be warning signs of a possible problematic case. Frequently, transgender women come to the office with previous rhinoplasties, and the most common complaints include high radix, sloping dorsum, broad osseous vault, inverted "V" deformity, over-rotated nasal tip, and excessive nostril reduction. In these revision, cases are imperative to explain to the patient the goals of the surgery: improve and reconstruct as much as possible.

SURGICAL TECHNIQUE
Marking and Pre-operative Infiltration

Marking the skin is a subjective and personal way to reference the important landmarks in rhinoplasty. Just mark the important points, because drawing too much may alter nose assessment. Basic drawing lines are the starting hump point, keystone point, anterior septal prominence point, dorsum desire line, and lateral osteotomies (**Fig. 1**A). The dorsum desire line is marked with the author's "rule of thumb": apply the width of the thumb (~25 mm) in the nasofacial groove and mark just above the thumb, then draw a line from the starting hump point, passing the "thumb line," and

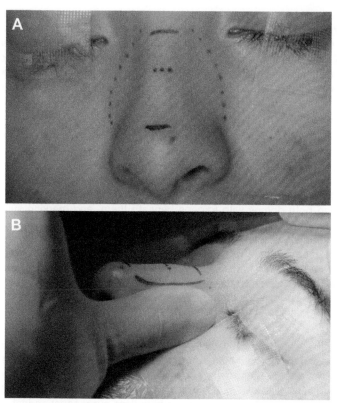

Fig. 1. Basic marking. (*A*) From top to bottom: Starting hump point, keystone point, and anterior septal prominence point. (*B*) The dorsum desire line is marked with the author's "rule of thumb".

ending at the anterior septal prominence (see **Fig. 1**B). Leaving the dorsum height at ~25 mm (measured at the nasofacial groove) it's esthetically appropriate for almost all patients.

After marking, infiltrate the nose with tumescent preparation: 1 vial of 50 mL of lidocaine 2%, epinephrine (lidocaine 20 mg/epinephrine 0.005 mg/1 mL) + 0.5 mL of pure epinephrine + 50 mL saline solution 0.9%. Infiltrate incision sites, osteotomies, and avoid infiltration at dorsum (it may distort dorsal height appreciation). Patient must be in semi-fowler position, with an ice pack on his or her face and request the anesthesiologist to maintain the mean arterial pressure at 60, wait about 15 to 20 mins of latency. The surgeon may perform turbinate reduction or any other small procedures necessary during the wait.

Approach

The author's first choice for feminization rhinoplasty is by a closed approach, via marginal incisions, and only in secondary or difficult cases, the surgery may be converted to an external approach if necessary. In the case of an external approach, the author has found better camouflaging of the incision scarring with a "W" pattern instead of an inverted "V," although there is no difference in the comparative study of Ihvan.[8]

Incisions in the closed approach start at the lateral columellar groove, then the inferior border of the lateral crus, avoid extending far away from the distal third of the lateral crus because there are vessels that may cause bleeding. The author's preferred starting point of dissection is the middle third of the lateral crus in a subperichondrial plane (if possible) to dissect all the surface, after that, dissecting the internal wall of the medial crus upward to the dome until joining both incisions at the end with scissors.

Inferior Lateral Cartilages Exposure

After exposing the inferior lateral cartilages (ILCs), it's helpful to loop reins at the domes with any kind of sutures, this helps for maneuvering the ILC instead of using hooks (**Fig. 2**A). The next step is to free the intercrural ligaments and Pitanguy Ligament just enough for good visualization of the anterior septal angle (ASA) and to gain mobility of the lateral crus (see **Fig. 2**B) and then to perform a dome symmetry test, elevating both domes with forceps beneath them, and marking symmetrically the desired new domes[9] (see **Fig. 2**C).

Cephalic trimming of lateral crus is helpful before approaching dorsum because it gives more space to maneuver in a closed approach. Leave intact about 7 mm of the lateral crura measured at the middle portion, just at the peak of the caudal border, and leave 5–6 mm at the domes. The trimming must be completed in a straight line, avoiding a curve pattern. It's important to save the trimmed cartilages, as later they will help as camouflage or Onlay dome grafts.

Dorsum Dissection

The starting point to access the dorsum is easily identified by applying caudal traction of the reins and then to enter with scissors just in the midline at the caudal point of upper lateral cartilages (ULCs) (**Fig. 3**A) and then to proceed to create a pocket just large enough for the instruments, dissecting in a bloodless supraperichondrial plane (sub-SMAS) and preserving the vertical scroll ligament. Separate just enough for adequate visualization.[10] Not preserving vertical scroll ligament results in bleeding. Dissecting sub-SMAS in the dorsum is essential to avoid edema and helps to achieve a better healing process. After the creation of the dorsal pocket, the periosteum is elevated just above the bony hump, preserving the rest over the nasal bones to avoid instability during osteotomies.

Hump Reduction

The "split hump reduction" technique (Daniel and Pálházi,2018)[11] involves removing the bony component first, followed by cartilage reduction after splitting off and

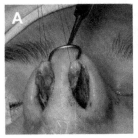
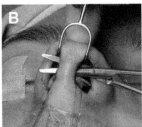
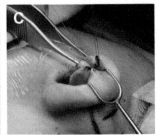

Fig. 2. Exposure of inferior lateral cartilages. (*A*) Reins placed at domes for maneuvering. (*B*) Lobular ligaments loosening. (*C*) dome symmetry test, elevating both domes with forceps beneath them, and marking symmetrically the desired new domes.

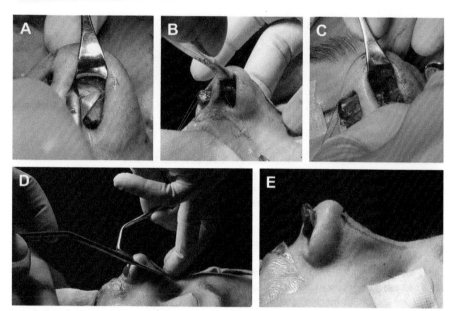

Fig. 3. Hump reduction. (*A*) Supraperichondrial dorsum dissection. (*B*) Bony hump reduction with rasp. (*C*) Superior lateral cartilage splitting from the septum. (*D*) Septal trimming direction toward the finger touching outside. (*E*) Dorsum desired line.

preserving the ULC. I suggest do not perform "en bloc" hump reduction, as it raises the possibility of an open roof deformity because it removes the underlying ULCs.[11,12]

By this point, the nasal septum and the cartilaginous vault are intact, which gives stability to the septal framework while rasping the bony hump. Rasping must be done in fast movements and not forced toward the face of the patient, as it may cause edema and inadvertent disruption of the keystone area (see **Fig. 3**B); it is necessary to maintain a perpendicular position of the rasp; this helps to avoid uneven shortening of either nasal bones. Continue rasping until the ideal dorsal height based on the previous marking is reached. Bony hump reduction must be done delicately with both hands, alternating palpating and rasping. Avoid pinching the skin toward the instruments. During the bony hump reduction, the cartilaginous vault must be intact, as well as the septum for added structural security.

Dorsal cartilage reduction begins with first exposing the ASA and approaching the intraseptal space via the subperichondrial plane bilaterally. The easiest way to find the plane of dissection is with electro-cautery touches to the septal perichondrium. Dissecting only one side of the septum perichondrium may result in traction forces to the contralateral side. Expose all the caudal septal border to the anterior nasal spine (ANS) then elevate the subperichondrial plane beneath ULC for further splitting from the septum with scissors or a blade (see **Fig. 3**C). Once the septum is separated from the ULCs, the author's maneuver is to introduce to the dorsum an Aufricht nasal retractor and externally touch the bony dorsum with a free finger, so the dorsal septal trimming direction, starting at the ASA, is toward the finger touching outside (see **Fig. 3**D).

The trimmed dorsal cartilage must be adequately calculated in relation to the ideal cartilage height (see **Fig. 3**E), as this could be used as a potential graft (especially in big cartilage humps). Preserve if possible the integrity of the complete septal cartilage.

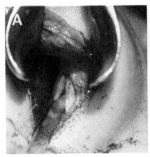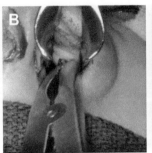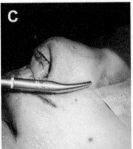

Fig. 4. Pyriform aperture exposure. (*A*) Dissection of pyriform aperture above the head of inferior turbinate. (*B*) Wedge resection. (*C*) Prominent maxillary ascendant process, a near-complete osteotomy can be performed using the bone Rongeur.

Osteotomies

Using a micro-electrocoagulation needle, a mucosal incision is made just above the head of the inferior turbinate at the level of the pyriform aperture. This avoids Webster's triangle collapse and prevents possible bleeding vessels that can be transected with a traditional vestibular incision. The next step is dissecting 5 mm inner and outer walls of the pyriform aperture (**Fig. 4**A), it's important to maintain intact the periosteum in the upper two-thirds of the maxillary ascending process, this helps to maintain bones attached and will help for a better healing stabilization process.

After exposing the piriform aperture above the turbinate, using bone cutting forceps (Beyer bone Rongeur), a bilateral wedge of bone at the frontal process of the maxilla is removed (see **Fig. 4**B).[13,14] The length of the wedge resection varies depending on the objective of the surgery and the anatomy itself. When treating a very high or prominent maxillary ascendant process, a near-complete lateral osteotomy can be performed using the bone Rongeur (see Fig. 4C). In low dorsums, just little wedge resection (3–5 mm) is advised. When treating a deviated nasal pyramid, the asymmetrical wedge resection is performed, being wider on the contralateral side of the deviation or at the longer nasal side. The wedge resection in all cases will help to firmly mount the osteotome without slipping and, in the author's opinion, will create a smooth and less traumatic travel of the osteotome. In addition, this maneuver prevents the collapse of the internal nasal valve by the medialized maxillary ascendant process after osteotomies.

The osteotomy trajectory in all cases is high-low-high.[15] Beginning above the head of the inferior turbinate and finishing just above of the boundary mark of the starting point of the hump. Almost all the cases do not require medial, or oblique medial osteotomies, and just joining both lateral osteotomies will be enough. Medial-oblique osteotomies are performed in very wide bony dorsums. Transverse osteotomies are performed with an endonasal transverse saw to connect lateral osteotomies and release bony mobilization. After lateral osteotomies, dorsum may elevate a few millimeters because of the in-fracture of the nasal sidewalls, including the septal cartilage, so it's important to review the desired dorsum height. After osteotomies, septum deviation may be corrected by itself just a little bit by gaining upward space.

Regarding breathing issues after osteotomies with this technique are unexpected because are not performed at the vestibular area, and the wedge resected bone will not obstruct the airway.

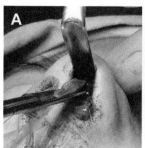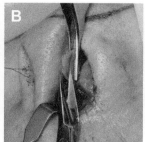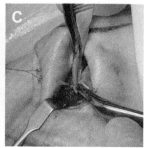

Fig. 5. Septal contouring technique. (*A*) Septal hump reduction. (*B*) Trimming of anterior septal angle. (*C*) Contouring of septal caudal border.

Septoplasty

In feminization rhinoplasty is frequent to deal with tension noses with large septal cartilages, the author approach is a "septal contouring technique," and this must be performed before the decision to harvest cartilage from the central septum. The cartilage harvested during these steps may be enough. The first step is during the septal hump reduction, then trimming the septal caudal border and ASA (**Fig. 5**). In case the septal graft harvested during the split hump reduction is sufficient, and no functional septal deviations need to be corrected, no further septal dissection is needed. If an excessive caudal septal cartilage is present, it could be trimmed to free tension on the nasolabial angle and will improve the columellar show in a tension nose and obtain a more natural appearance.[16] Generally, a prominent ANS coexists, so can be excised too. The cartilage trimmed will be saved as a graft after septal contouring proceeds to correct cartilage and bony deviations.

The author noticed that starting a rhinoplasty with the septoplasty may cause further problems at the end. When first addressing septal deviations and rushing to harvest the septal graft, we may lose the perception of the "L" strut, especially if a large amount of septal cartilage is removed or when the vomer and perpendicular plate are resected. At first, we may think that we performed a great septoplasty, but when reducing the dorsum cartilage, the "L" strut will be compromised noticing that we can't lower the dorsum anymore because of the cartilage left behind, and the ideal dorsum height will be unavailable. The next problem is the osteotomies, If we perform the septoplasty first and resect a large septal bone, we are removing the buttress just below the bony vault, so afterward, osteotomies may destabilize the dorsum and risk saddle nose deformity. In addition, many times the septum gets in the midline just after the osteotomies, and it is not necessary to resect more tissue. This is the same for preservation dorsum techniques. Therefore, leaving the septal work at the end, the 10 to 15 mm "L" strut will not be altered or compromised.

Cartilaginous Vault Repair

In a closed approach, it may seem a challenge to repair the cartilaginous vault but using the correct instruments may simplify the process (**Fig. 6**). Depending on the case, the closure may be simple suturing, autospreader flaps, or spreader grafts. When small humps are removed, it's enough to close the dorsum with simple suturing with 5-0 PDS. With larger humps, the excess of ULC will be rotated inward for creating autospreader flaps and secured with 5-0 PDS. Spreader grafts are used only in dorsal cartilaginous deviations and secondary cases with collapsed ULC or inverted "V" deformity.

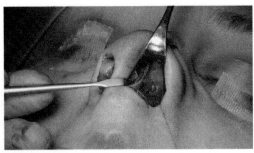

Fig. 6. Cartilaginous vault repair with auto-spreaders. Small retractors easily expose the dorsum in a closed approach.

Nasal Tip Work

The next step is to define and change the orientation of domes and lateral crus. This is achieved by hemi-transdomal suture published by Gruber and colleagues (2010)[17,18] and described as cephalic dome suture by Cakir and Dogan (2013).[19] It consists of placing a 5-0 PDS suture just above the ideal dome and joining cephalic borders of the medial and lateral crus. Modified hemi-transdomal sutures by Dogan (2020)[20] describe placing three sutures 1 mm to each other, the proximal suture to the dome is tight, and the distal sutures are loose, thus creating a triangular shape between medial and lateral crus and correcting the resting angle (**Fig. 7**). The concept of resting angle described by Cakir and colleagues (2012)[21] consists in creating a divergence angle of 100° between the cephalic border of lateral crus and the ULC.

Tip support, rotation, and projection are stabilized with an anterior nasal septal angle (ANSA) extension graft as described by Neves (2020).[22] The advantage of this technique is that a large graft is not required and will support the tip position in the long term and without the stiffness caused by a traditional septal extension graft (**Fig. 8**). The dimensions of the graft are about 10 to 15 mm long, 3–5 mm width at the anterior aspect, and 5–8 mm at the posterior aspect and trapezoid crafted.[22] The ANSA graft must be just at the midline, so identifying caudal septal laterality is the first step before placing the graft. The ANSA graft is secured to the septum with 5-0 PDS or Prolene, anchoring both cephalic and caudal borders of the graft and mattress sutures at the center. The projection length of the graft out of the ASA

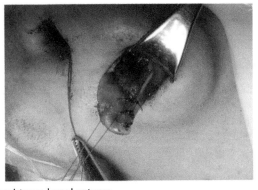

Fig. 7. Modified hemi-transdomal sutures.

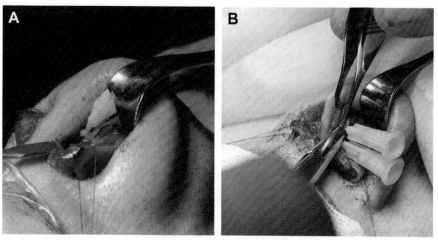

Fig. 8. Anterior nasal septal angle graft. (*A*) Closed approach. (*B*) Open approach.

depends on the desired result but ranges between 5 to 10 mm. The proposed angulation of the graft by Neves (2020)[22] is 130° in relation to the dorsum. In transgender secondary rhinoplasties, over-rotated and small nasal tips are a frequent find because of previous excessive caudal border resection, the author uses an angle of 160° to 180° to correct overrotation and project the ANSA graft 10 mm. The next step is to secure the new domes to the ANSA graft placing 5-0 PDS sutures passing through the lateral crus near the domes without suturing the medial crus; this will create an additional external rotation at the resting angle (**Fig. 9**).

If excessive bending of the medial crus is observed, or hanging columella is present, perform a medial crus overlap procedure[9]: transect the medial crus, undermine the distal aspect, overlap both ends, and then secure with 5-0 PDS (**Fig. 10**D–F). If bending of the lateral crus is present, transect it at the distal lateral third, and overlap the ends (see Fig. 10A–C), Dogan (2020)[20] explains that leaving the transected lateral

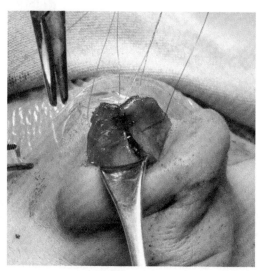

Fig. 9. Securing the new domes to the ANSA graft and opening the resting angle.

crus without suturing will not affect the results because now the tip is supported by the ANSA graft, not by the lateral crus. The author has confirmed this in his own experience, in performing unilateral transection of lateral crus without suturing, the transected side always resulted in a better appearance without pinching, instead of the sutured one or if it wasn't transected. Leaving the healing process by itself of the transected lateral crus causes less traction forces or stiffness that could produce asymmetry or pinching. However, bear in mind that there must be an overlap in undermining one end for free movement. Medial and lateral crus overlap procedures are performed frequently in feminization rhinoplasty, as they deproject the nasal tip. Lateral crural overlay is an excellent technique to adjust the projection and rotation of the nasal tip without compromising the structural integrity of the external nasal valve.[23]

For tip support, an ANSA graft is enough, and no further columellar strut is required, instead restructuring the medial crus with sutures. Join the posterior borders of the intermediate crus to the ANSA graft with a spanning suture (**Fig. 11**A–C); this will open the divergence angle of the medial crus, causing external rotation of the caudal borders and creating an open appearance of the infratip. Once getting the desired divergence angle, excess of medial crus can be trimmed and reshaped to a columellar break. Only in cases where the medial crus are weak or mutilated, a columellar strut with an angled shape is used (see **Fig. 11**D–F). Nasal tip is finalized by placing trimmed cephalic border of lateral crus as Onlay graft over the new domes, which will help to smooth and avoid sharp edges at the tip (**Fig. 12**).

Incision Closure

Close marginal incisions with resorbable sutures as 5-0 monocryl and secure septal mucosa with transeptal continuous suturing in all the anterior septum, which is enough to avoid septal hematomas and spare intranasal splints, and irrigate with a cold tumescent solution inside the osteotomies incisions and leave them open.

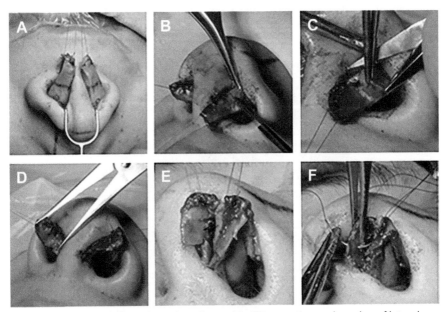

Fig. 10. Deprojecting inferior lateral cartilages. (*A–C*) Transection and overlap of lateral crus. Note that the ends are not secured. (*D–F*) medial crus overlap procedure.

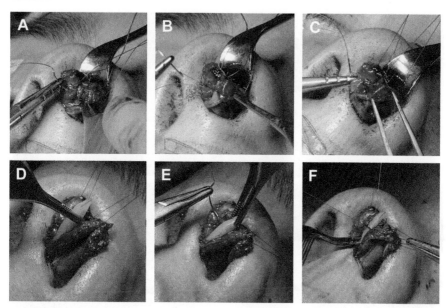

Fig. 11. Restructure of the intermediate and medial crus with the opening of divergence angle. (*A–C*) Spanning sutures. (*D–F*) Placing columellar strut if required.

Alar Base Reduction

The author's philosophy about alar base reduction is only to do it if it's completely necessary. If after 6 to 12 months, the alar base does not match the rhinoplasty results or the patient has complaints about it; it can be performed in the office and with the certainty of the results obtained overall. Alar base reduction in feminization rhinoplasty must be conservative enough, as this could be a surgical stigma, in which the surgeon with the idea to "feminize" the nose, resects a lot of the alar base and creates small noses that look awkward.

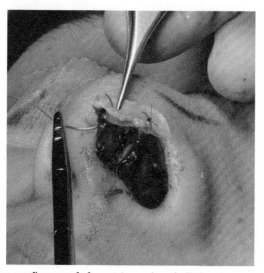

Fig. 12. Onlay tip camouflage graft from trimmed cephalic border.

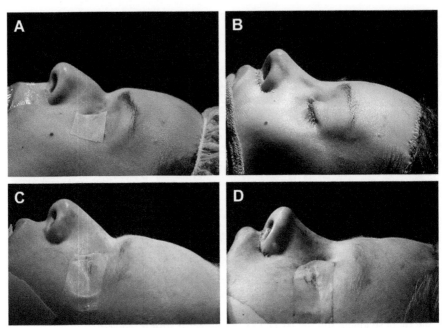

Fig. 13. Frontal bone remodeling, hairline advancement, lip lift, and feminization rhinoplasty. (*A and B*) Patient 1 before and after. (*C and D*) Patient 2 before and after.

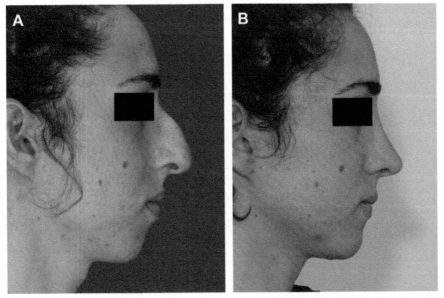

Fig. 14. Feminization rhinoplasty, chin advancement, and thyroid angle chondroplasty. (*A*) before. (*B*) After.

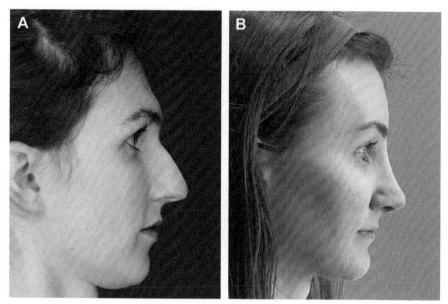

Fig. 15. Feminization rhinoplasty, frontal bone remodeling, chin advancement, and thyroid angle chondroplasty. (*A*) Before. (*B*) After.

The author's preference for alar base reduction is to use the micro-electrocoagulation tip to resect the alar base without bleeding; the healing process is excellent; and the author has never found any issue. After marking the excess of alar flaring or nasal sill, the pattern of the incisions may be a spindle shape for sill excess or semilunar for flaring or a combination of both. Sill incision must be kept medial to the long axis of the nostril; resecting vestibular skin (lateral to the long axis of nostril) will cause a "Q" or teardrop deformity[24] and then close the incisions with 5-0 vicryl buried subcutaneous sutures and skin with 5-0 plastic monocryl.

SUMMARY

Surgical philosophy and concepts have changed a lot in recent years, and what was previously widely unanimously accepted to be true is now questioned. Surgeons defy the teachings and create new techniques, relive old ones, and use new technology. The exchange of ideas and artistry is now easy with social media and webinars all around which has evolved rhinoplasty.

Tip surgery has become more simple and minimalist than years before. The past use of large bulky grafts on the tip has resulted in a lot of revision cases taking out the grafts over the passing years, showing us we need to go in another direction. Preservation is the tendency now, and not just for osteocartilaginous vault descent techniques (push or let down), but preserving ligaments, septal cartilage and destroying as little as possible. Reorientation and tension-free techniques of the alar cartilages have gained popularity because of the natural appearance of the results. All these new concepts positively impact feminization rhinoplasty. We achieve more natural results, and the possibility of reducing the size of the nose in all dimensions is of paramount importance in the transgender woman.[25]

Feminization rhinoplasty uses the same techniques as cisgender rhinoplasty, but there is an additional impact in the improvement of a patient's quality of life after rhinoplasty. Therefore, implementation of transgender health education is important in all levels, and we need to be prepared to perform gender-affirming surgery as the incidence of patients present for gender-affirming surgeries is growing.[26]

Treating transgender patients needs a complete facial analysis and will rarely benefit from only one procedure to feminize facial features. For superior results, it's recommended to offer frontal bone remodeling and rhinoplasty at a minimum (**Figs. 13–15**). Creating a smooth dorsal line from the forehead to the nasal tip, proper nasofrontal angle and nasolabial angle is of critical importance.[27] With these two procedures, almost all patients improve facial gender dysphoria. Bellinga and colleagues (2017)[28] have published that 75% of feminization rhinoplasty is combined with forehead reconstruction. This is the highest number of feminization rhinoplasties published by 2016 with 200 patients. By this time, this number must be superior and hope to have a new research paper by their group soon.

Facial feminization surgery significantly improves the quality of life for transgender women and simultaneously affords the rhinoplasty surgeon the chance to apply the limits of his or her skills to the great benefit of the patient.[29]

DISCLOSURE

The author has nothing to disclose.

ACKNOWLEDGMENTS

Stacy Barr Velasco, MA, for her help editing this chapter. Jesús Báez-Pérez, photographer, for the shots and being my dad. Fernando Guzmán-Lozano, MD, teacher, uncle, and great partner in surgery. Nancy Medina, MD, for her comprehensive love. Leonor Márquez-Amezcua, for being such a lovely mom. Julie and Leo for being so wonderful kids. Elsa Lepe, For her collaboration on my team, and her fight for transgender rights.

REFERENCES

1. Morrison SD, Capitán-Cañadas F, Sánchez-García A, et al. Prospective quality-of-life outcomes after facial feminization surgery: an international multicenter study. Plast Reconstr Surg 2020;145:1499–509.
2. Morrison S, Vyas KS, Gast KM, et al. Facial feminization: systematic review of the literature. Plast Reconstr Surg 2016;137:1759–70.
3. JU Berli, Loyo M. Gender-confirming rhinoplasty. Facial Plast Surg Clin N Am 2019;27:251–60.
4. Ousterhout DK. Feminization of the forehead: contour changing to improve female aesthetics. Plast Reconstr Surg 1987;79:701–13.
5. Hamidi O, Davidge-Pitts CJ. Transfeminine hormone therapy. Endocrinol Metab Clin N Am 2019;48:341–55.
6. Callen AL, Badiee RK, Phelps A, et al. Facial feminization surgery: key CT findings for preoperative planning and postoperative evaluation. AJR Am J Roentgenol 2021;217:709–17.
7. Bashiri-Bawil M, Rahavi-Ezabadi S, Sadeghi M, et al. Preoperative computer simulation in rhinoplasty using previous postoperative images. Facial Plast Surg Aesthet Med 2020;22:406–11.
8. Ihvan O, Seneldir L, Naiboglu B, et al. Comparative columellar scar analysis between W incisions and inverted-V incision in open technique nasal surgery. Indian J Otolaryngol Head Neck Surg 2018;70:231–4.

9. Çakır B. Aesthetic septorhinoplasty. In: Chapter 13 results. Switzerland: Springer; 2016. p. 195.
10. Neves JC, Zholtikov V, Çakır B. Rhinoplasty dissection planes (subcutaneous, sub-SMAS, supra-perichondral, and sub-perichondral) and soft tissues management. Facial Plast Surg 2021;37:2–11.
11. Daniel RK, Palhazi P. Rhinoplasty an anatomical and clinical atlas. In: Chapter 3 Osseocartilaginous vault. Switzerland: Springer; 2018. p. 132–3.
12. Palhazi P, Daniel RK, Kosins AM. The osseocartilaginous vault of the nose: anatomy and surgical observations. Aesthet Surg J 2015;35:242–51.
13. Patel PN, Abdelwahab M, Most SP. A review and modification of dorsal preservation rhinoplasty techniques. Facial Plast Surg Aesthet Med 2020;22:71–9.
14. Lothrop O. An operation for correcting the aquiline nasal deformity; the use of new instrument; report of a case. Boston Med Surg J 1914;170:835–7.
15. Azizzadeh B, Reilly M. Dorsal hump reduction and osteotomies. Clin Plast Surg 2016;43:47–58.
16. Kantas IV, Papadakis CE, Balatsouras DG, et al. Functional tension nose as a cause of nasal airway obstruction. Auris Nasus Larynx 2007;34:313–7.
17. Gruber RP, Chang E, Buchanan E. Suture techniques in rhinoplasty. Clin Plast Surg 2010;37:231–43.
18. Dosanjh AS, Hsu C, Gruber RP. The hemitransdomal suture for narrowing the nasal tip. Ann Plast Surg 2010;64:708–12.
19. Çakır B, Dogan T, Oreroglu AR, et al. Rhinoplasty: surface aesthetics and surgical techniques. Aesthet Surg J 2013;33:363–75.
20. Dogan T. Teorhinoplasty. In: Surgical technique. Istanbul: Ofset Yapimevi; 2020. p. 94–6.
21. Çakır B, Oreroglu AR, Daniel RK. Surface aesthetics in tip rhinoplasty: a step-by-step guide. Aesthet Surg J 2014;34:941–55.
22. Neves JC, Tagle DA. Lateral crura control in nasal tip plasty: cephalic oblique domal suture, 7x suture and ansa banner. Ann Plast Reconstr Surg 2020;4:1059.
23. Insalaco L, Rashes ER, Rubin SJ, et al. Association of lateral crural overlay technique with strength of the lower lateral cartilages. JAMA Facial Plast Surg 2017; 19:510–5.
24. Cobo R, Conderman CP, Kridel RW. Ethnic considerations in facial plastic surgery. In: Chapter 14 Approach to the nasal base in patients of African descent. New York: Thieme Publishers; 2016. p. 150.
25. Spiegel JH. Considerations in feminization rhinoplasty. Facial Plast Surg 2020; 36:53–6.
26. Canner JK, Harfouch O, Kodadek LM, et al. Temporal trends in gender-affirming surgery among transgender patients in the united states. JAMA Surg 2018;153: 609–16.
27. Deschamps-Braly JC. Facial gender confirmation surgery facial feminization surgery and facial masculinization surgery. Clin Plast Surg 2018;45:323–31.
28. Bellinga RJ, Capitan L, Simon D, et al. Technical and clinical considerations for facial feminization surgery with rhinoplasty and related procedures. JAMA Facial Plast Surg 2017;19:175–81.
29. Spiegel JH. Rhinoplasty as a significant component of facial feminization and beautification. JAMA Facial Plast Surg 2017;19:181–2.

Cheek Augmentation in Gender-Affirming Facial Surgery

Jeffrey S. Jumaily, MD

KEYWORDS

- Gender-affirming facial surgery • Cheek • Augmentation • Alloplastic cheek implants
- Fat grafting

KEY POINTS

- High cheekbones and full malar area is considered a desired feminine feature and therefore is an important component of gender-affirming facial surgery.
- Fillers are customizable and reversible and have minimal recovery but are not preferred because of the need for maintenance and cost.
- Fat grafting has many desirable characteristics, such as abundance, customizability, biocompatibility, and relative low cost, but long-term data of longevity are lacking.
- Alloplastic implants offer predictable augmentation volume, easy of placement, relatively low cost, and availability of various shapes and sizes. However, alloplastic implants carry the risk of infection, malposition, asymmetry, and visibility in thin-skinned patients.

The malar area is considered to be one of the most important regions to an attractive and youthful face. Beauty trends have changed over the decades, and current trends in beauty as seen in many fashion and other models is high cheekbones with full cheeks. This trend seems to be consistent across the globe and its many ethnicities. A study of composite photographs of white and Japanese women reported that women were rated higher if they had higher cheekbones, suggesting that various ethnicities share similar beauty standards.[1]

Cheeks that have the right amount of definition and volume are essential for a balanced midface. The midface, which is centered on the prominent midline structure of the nose, and also the chin prominence, requires the malar and zygoma regions to have volume and shape to balance the nose and chin, and also to support the lower-lid structure. Constantinides and colleagues[2] suggested that the golden ratio (Φ) applies to the malar area in the form of a golden rectangle of the malar eminence that is bordered superiorly by a line drawn at the lower border of the arc of the eyebrows, laterally at the lateral canthi and inferiorly by a line between the alar rims (**Fig. 1**).

No disclosures.
Jeffrey Jumaily Facial Plastic Surgery, 5757 Wilshire Boulevard PR2, Los Angeles, CA 90036, USA
E-mail address: info@drjumaily.com

Anatomically, the malar region is formed by skin, adipose tissue, facial muscles in the SMAS (superficial musculoaponeurotic system), and the underlying bone. These anatomic layers are subject to all the usual changes of life, including aging, sun exposure, animation, gravity, weight changes, immune and health conditions, nutrition, smoking, genetics, and others. The fat compartments of the malar area deserve some careful attention, and they have been studied extensively. There are superficial and deep fat compartments in the face. The superficial midfacial fat compartments include the infraorbital fat, superficial medial cheek fat, and nasolabial fat. The deep midfacial fat compartments include the medial and lateral suborbicularis oculi fat, the deep medial cheek fat, which can be further divided into medial and lateral parts, and the medial portion of the buccal fat pad.[3]

Ousterhout[4] and Spiegel[5] and others have done extensive work in comparing the surgical anatomy of men and women. Lambros and Amos[6] compared 3-dimensional photographs of men and woman of various ages. They found that male faces are generally larger. They downsized the pictures by 8.4% to equalize the size, surface area, and other measurements. After controlling for the size, they noted that men have flatter anterior maxilla and smaller cheeks, among other differences. Much anatomic and clinical work in the literature focuses on the effect of aging on the cheek anatomy. Although many gender-affirming surgery patients have signs of aging, the focus for this publication is to discuss the difference between the common male cheek anatomy and the desired ideal feminine appearance and how to achieve it. In other words, in the spectrum of volume restoration versus volume enhancement, in the author's experience, gender-affirming surgery patients often want volume enhancement at all ages rather than restoration of their younger appearance.

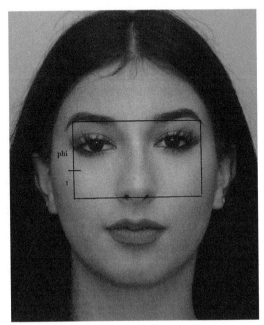

Fig. 1. The golden ratio (*phi*) applies to the malar area in the form of a golden rectangle of the malar eminence that is bordered superiorly by a line drawn at the lower border of the arc of the eyebrows, laterally at the lateral canthi and inferiorly by a line between the alar rims.

Like any facial aesthetic endeavor, careful evaluation and analysis of the face are paramount. Gender-affirming surgery patients tend to be well informed, to be well researched, and sometimes have a precise idea of what they want. The vast majority would like more feminine cheeks. The surgeon's goal is to give the patient defined high cheeks with appropriate volume in the context of the patient's goals. Often, the patients will ask for "aggressive" and "transformative" rather than subtle results. The surgeon has to navigate the patient's wishes and preconceptions and reconcile them with the limitations of the technique, the surgeon's own aesthetic judgment, and the surgeon's ability.

TECHNIQUES

Broadly, cheek augmentation and enhancement can be done nonsurgically with injectable fillers or surgically with autologous fat transfer, alloplastic implants, or lifting techniques. The lifting techniques, including midface lift and deep plane facelift, are discussed extensively in the literature and can be combined with other filling techniques based on the "lift-and-fill" mantra.[7] Lifting techniques are outside the scope of this article. The author focuses the discussion on comparing autologous fat transfer with alloplastic implants because these are the workhorses of cheek enhancement in gender-confirming surgery patients.

INJECTABLE FILLERS

Fillers are a great option for many patients and is widely used for malar enhancement by practitioners of all subspecialties. Hyaluronic acid (HA) fillers are safe and effective in the cheek area. Fillers are popular in the general population owing to heir safety, quick recovery, good results, and low upfront cost. Many of the author's patients experiment with fillers in their lips and occasionally cheeks before considering gender-affirming surgery. However, they quickly dismiss it as a long-term solution, as it requires frequent maintenance. In addition, they desire a significant augmentation that requires a higher volume of HA fillers, which can get costly quickly with maintenance and frequent doctor visits. In addition, they are planning a large facial surgery with a long recovery, so down time and upfront cost are less of a hurdle. Last, large-volume augmentation with fillers can be associated with unnatural appearance, skin changes, and migration. Therefore, HA filler cheek augmentation is a small part of the author's gender-affirming surgery practice. For full discussion of filler usage and technique, the reader is encouraged to seek the numerous texts and articles and live demonstrations from experienced practitioners that are widely available.

AUTOLOGOUS FAT GRAFTING

Fat transfer has a long history extending over a century.[8,9] However, the popularity of fat transfer increased as the popularity of liposuction increased.[10] Fat transfer remains controversial as to whether it has long-term survival.[11] There is a lack of high-quality objective studies to evaluate whether transplanted fat actually persists over time. However, fat is the closest we have to the ideal augmentation material owing to its availability, ease of harvest, biocompatibility, and noncarcinogenicity.

Donor Site Location

There are many reports in the literature that discuss the best donor site. However, no quality studies exist that can support use of one site over another.[10] Rohrich and colleagues[12] examined various fat samples using spectrometry and found them to be equivalent. In the author's experience, the medial thighs are safe, have available fat, and are less painful and less fibrous than abdominal fat. The abdomen is the second site if the medial thighs are not suitable for any reason. The author has also used the buccal fat pad if a simultaneous procedure is planned.

Aspiration Methods

Several techniques have been proposed to harvest fat, including direct excision, blunt aspiration, and sharp aspiration. Aspiration is still the most popular method, but consensus is missing owing to conflicting evidence.[10] In a rat model, direct excision appears to have the best survival.[13] There is some consensus that manual aspiration with a 10-cc syringe and low vacuum pressure are preferred. The size of cannula is not agreed on, but a 3-mm cannula is preferred by some surgeons. In the author's practice, he uses a 10-cc syringe with 2 to 3 cc of plunger pull to aspirate through a 3-mm blunt cannula after infiltration of the area with a tumescent solution that includes a mixture of 50 mL 2% lidocaine, 1 mL epinephrine (1:1000), in 1 L of lactated Ringer solution.

Washing and Centrifugation

There is debate as to whether washing the grafts improves graft survival. Investigators have presented evidence that washing the fat with sterile water, Cariel solution, or Ringer may improve graft survival, but no consensus exists.[10] There is consensus that the fat should be separated by centrifuge or gravity to remove the top oil layer and the bottom blood and tumescent layer, which is what the author does at his practice.

Exposure to Air or Growth Factors

At the author's practice, they try to minimize exposure to air, as there is evidence that it can increase cell lysis.[14]

There are studies that showed improved cell survival with the addition of insulin, nutrient media, hormones, and others, but the clinical evidence is not strong enough to encourage its use.[10] In the author's practice, they do not use a mix any growth factors with the fat. They must keep a close eye on the new evidence regarding adipocyte-derived stem cells, as it appears promising.

Surgical Technique

Once the fat is harvested and separated, it is time to place it. It was suggested that fat cells need to be within 2 mm of arterial supply to survive.[15] Several types and sizes of cannulas have been used from 17- to 14-gauge blunt cannulas and 2- to 3-mm cannulas as well.[10] A blunt-tipped cannula is preferred here to avoid bleeding and trauma. To maximize proximity to vascularized tissue, the fat is placed in small aliquots in tunnels created by the cannula in the "fanning" technique. Tunnel overlap should be minimized. The entry point of the cannula is done with an 18-gauge needle (**Figs. 2–4**).

It is important to note that fat grafting's long-term outcomes are poorly studied. There are several animal studies and clinical data, but few have adequate objective evidence to demonstrate true graft survival and growth. The community needs studies using technology that can quantify tissue volume, and surface volume can give us meaningful evidence as to whether the liposuctioned fat can truly survive in vivo in the long term.

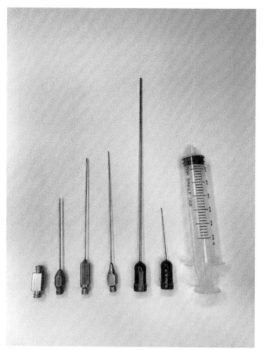

Fig. 2. Cannulas used in the fat harvest and injection process.

Complications

Lipoinjection is generally a very safe procedure. Several reports shed light on the possible rare complications. The main concern with any injection in the face is the possibility of fat emboli that can lead to occlusion of end organ vessels in the skin, brain, and eyes. Fat emboli leading to blindness, stroke, and even death have been reported,[16–21] especially with injections in the glabella, nasolabial folds, and periorbital areas. These are rare but should be discussed with the patient, and surgeons should keep these possibilities in mind during and after the procedure. More minor common complications are contour irregularities, hematoma, infection, and poor long-term fat survival.

ALLOPLASTIC CHEEK AUGMENTATION

Alloplastic midfacial implants can play a major role in the rejuvenation and enhancement of the midface. Although fillers and fat grafting offer soft tissue augmentation options, implants augment the underlying skeleton. The vertical height added by the implant has a lifting effect on the soft tissue, which can lead to improvement in the nasolabial folds in addition to augmenting the cheeks.[22] Lifting procedures combined with implants are much more effective, as the surgeon can drape the soft tissue on a more projected and enhanced skeleton. Other advantages of implants are their stable long-term outcomes, long-term cost-effectiveness, and quick recovery. Gender-affirming surgery patients often dislike any procedures that require repeated maintenance, such as fillers, making implants a good option.

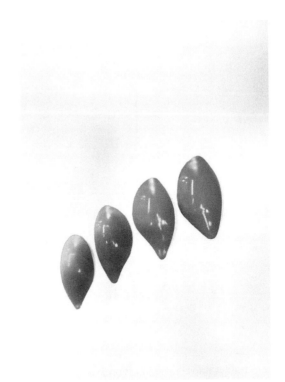

Fig. 3. Conform Terino Malar Shell sizers, from left to right: small, medium, large, and extralarge.

IMPLANT MATERIAL AND TYPES

Historically, nonfat, autologous tissue was used for augmentation, such as iliac crest, costal cartilage, auricular cartilage, split calvarial grafts, dermal grafts, and others.[2] The drawbacks included donor site morbidity, resorption, and difficulty of contouring and led to the search for the optimal alloplastic implant that is safe, noncarcinogenic, customizable, inexpensive, and that does not induce inflammatory or immunogenic reactions.

The common materials that are used and studied are silicone, polytetrafluoroethylene (PTFE) implants, and high-density polyethylene (HDPE). Silicone is a very commonly used facial implant in the chin, jaw, midface, and upper face. There is no tissue ingrowth, and the body forms a capsule around it; hence, it can be easily removed if needed. It can be easily carved intraoperatively or customized. Several studies highlighted its safety and patient satisfaction.[23–26] Implants are manufactured in various shapes, but the 2 general types are malar or submalar. Malar implants are used for patients who need augmentation in the zygoma to create more lateral projection and highlight but have normal midface soft tissue volume. Submalar implants are designed to augment the cheek soft tissue near malar eminence if the patient has adequate zygoma projection. The author finds the latter to be more common and uses more submalar implants than malar implants. For both zygoma and soft tissue–deficient patients, a combined or custom implant may be required.

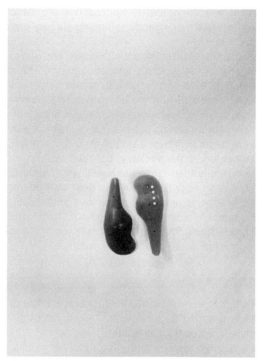

Fig. 4. Binder submalar implants sizers.

PTFE used in facial surgery was produced under the brand names Proplast and Gor-Tex. Proplast was taken off the market owing to delamination under shear stress. Gor-Tex is expandedPTFE, which is a porous material that allows limited fibrovascular ingrowth, which makes it slightly harder to remove.[2] It is a spongy material, that is customizable and does not induce reactions.

HDPE is a solid but flexible material produced under the brand name Medpor. It is a porous material that allows for soft tissue and limited bony in-growth.[2] Therefore, HDPE is difficult to remove after implantation. Several investigators have researched the stability of the implants over time. It was noted that a biofilm forms over the implant during infection, but this can be minimized with preimpregnation with antibiotics.[26] Another issue is that the tissue ingrowth through the pores stabilizes the implants in the soft tissue but not against bone, similar to silastic implant capsules.[27]

In the author's practice, silicone implants are preferred owing to familiarity and ease of removal, and anecdotal experience of many infected Medpor implants that are difficult to remove.

Surgical Technique

The first step is always a thorough facial evaluation, followed by a decision that is made with the patient to proceed with cheek augmentation. There are numerous ways to locate the malar eminence in order to decide the position of the implant and ensure symmetry.[2] In the author's practice, he uses the Prendergast and Schoenrock model, which bases the location of the malar eminence on a line drawn from the lateral canthus to the commissure, as the malar eminence is one-third from the canthus.[28] The implant position is then marked over the skin bilaterally to ensure symmetry. Although lower blepharoplasty approaches are described, an intraoral approach is preferred because many gender-affirming surgery patients do not require simultaneous blepharoplasty.[29]

After injection of local anesthesia in the anterior cheek and upper gingivobuccal sulcus, an incision is made in the mucosa and periosteum. The periosteum is then elevated over the anterior maxilla and zygoma to create a pocket in the desired location. Using a "no-touch" technique, the implant, which was preimpregnated with antibiotic solution, is placed in the pocket without contact with the teeth or oral mucosa. A polyglygolic acid guiding suture can be used to pull the tail in the lateral pocket, which can be tied in the temporal hairline over a button for 5 to 7 days. Fixation can be performed with a screw or suture. If the pocket is tight and mobility is minimal, fixation is not necessary. The incision is then closed in layers using absorbable sutures. Tape over the skin for 5 to 7 days is optional but can help with edema and immobilizing the implant. Systemic preoperative and postoperative antibiotics are used in the author's practice. It is debatable whether patients should take prophylactic antibiotics before future dental procedures. The author generally recommends them for the first year but without strong evidence to support this practice.

Complications

Midface implants, like any surgical procedure, are associated with postoperative edema and discomfort, but generally this is mild and lasts a few days. Eighty percent of edema usually resolves within 3 to 4 weeks.[22] However, other complications can occur, such as infection, malposition, asymmetry, extrusion, hematoma, seroma, fistula, persistent inflammatory reaction, and infraorbital nerve injury.[30] Infection rates are about 1%, and permanent nerve injury is quite rare. In the author's experience, an infection can develop up to 5 years after implantation presumably from bacteremia or acute rhinosinusitis, so patients are counseled to report any symptoms of erythema, pain, and edema over the implant area.

CLINICS CARE POINTS

- The malar eminence should be marked and symmetry is ensured prior to injection or implant placement.
- Despite the predictability, avoid overcorrecting with fat grafting to prevent overfilled cheeks appearance.
- If a cheek implant shows signs of infection, remove the implant and replace after the infection has resolved.

SUMMARY

Malar augmentation can lead to significant enhancement and feminization of the cheek area. A detailed patient evaluation is required to determine the need and extent of the augmentation required. The patient should be counseled on the available options, including autologous fat transfer and the various alloplastic implant and injectable fillers. Autologous fat is a great, albeit slightly unpredictable procedure for augmentation. Further studies are needed to determine how much fat survives using the known methods. This knowledge can help surgeons decide if this procedure is the best choice for their patients. Alloplastic implants have excellent long-term outcomes and reliability and are reversible. The risk of infection and need for removal should be discussed with the patient. Regardless of the augmentation method or material used, cheek augmentation is a safe and effective procedure that can help improve the patient's attractiveness and femininity.

REFERENCES

1. Perrett DI, May KA, Yoshokawa S. Facial shape and judgements of female attractiveness. Nature 1994;368:239–42.
2. Constantinides MS, Galli SK, Miller PJ, et al. Malar, submalar, and midfacial implants. Facial Plast Surg 2000;16(1):35–44.
3. Rohrich RJ, Avashia YJ. Savetsky IL Prediction of facial aging using the facial fat compartments. Plast Reconstr Surg 2021;147(1S-2):38S–42S.
4. Ousterhout DK. Feminization of the forehead: contour changing to improve female aesthetics. Plast Reconstr Surg 1987;79:701–13.
5. Spiegel JH. Facial feminization for the transgender patient. J Craniofac Surg 2019;30(5):1399–402.
6. Lambros V, Amos G. Facial Shape, Size, and Gender. Plast Reconstr Surg 2020; 146(5):1012–4.
7. Rohrich RJ, Ghavami A, Constantine FC, et al. Lift-and-fill facelift: integrating the fat compartments. Plast Reconstr Surg 2014;133:756e–67e.
8. Neuber F. Fetttransplantation. Zentrabl Chir 1893;22:66.
9. Miller CG. Cannula implants and review of implantation techniques in esthetic surgery. Chicago: Oak Press; 1926.
10. Kaufman MR. Autologous fat transfer for facial recontouring: is there science behind the art? Plast Reconstr Surg 2007;119:2287.
11. Calabria R. Fat grafting: fact or fiction? Aesthet Surg J 2005;25:55.
12. Rohrich RJ, Sorokin ES, Brown SA. In search of improved fat transfer viability: a quantitative analysis of the role of centrifugation and harvest site. Plast Reconstr Surg 2004;113:391.
13. Marques A, Brenda E, Saldiva PH, et al. Autologous fat grafts: a quantitative and morphometric study in rabbits. Scand J Plast Reconstr Surg Hand Surg 1994; 28:241.
14. Aboudib JHC, Cardoso de Castro C, Gradel J. Hand rejuvenescence by fat filling. Ann Plast Surg 1992;28:559.
15. Cook T, Nakra T, Shorr N, et al. Facial recontouring with autogenous fat. Facial Plast Surg 2004;20:145.
16. Feinendegen DL, Baumgartner RW, Vuadens P, et al. Autologous fat injection for soft tissue augmentation in the face: a safe procedure? Aesthetic Plast Surg 1998;22:163.
17. Dreizen NG, Framm L. Sudden unilateral visual loss after autologous fat injection into the glabellar area. Am J Ophthalmol 1989;107:85.
18. Egido JA, Arroyo R, Marcos A, et al. Middle cerebral artery embolism and unilateral visual loss after autologous fat injection into the glabellar area. Stroke 1993; 24:615.
19. Teimourian B. Blindness following fat injections. Plast Reconstr Surg 1988;82:361.
20. Thaunat O, Thaler F, Loirat P, et al. Cerebral fat embolism induced by facial fat injection. Plast Reconstr Surg 2004;113:2235.
21. Yoon SS, Chang DI, Chung KC. Acute fatal stroke immediately following autologous fat injection into the face. Neurology 2003;61:1151.
22. Dhir L, Binder W. Solid midfacial implants: when fillers are not enough. Facial Plast Surg 2016;32(5):480–7.

23. Costantine PD. Synthetic biomaterials for soft-tissue augmentation and replacement in the head and neck. Otolaryngol Clin North Am 1994;27:223–62.

24. Metzinger SE, McCollough G, Campbell JP, et al. Malar augmentation: a 5 year retrospective review of the silastic midfacial malar implant. Arch Otolaryngol Head Neck Surg 1999;125:980–7.

25. Ivy EJ, Lorenc P, Aston SJ. Malar augmentation with silicone implants. Plast Reconstr Surg 1995;96:63–8.

26. Sclafani AP, Thomas JR, Cox AJ, et al. Clinical and histologic response of subcutaneous expanded polytetrafluoroethylene (Gore-Tex) and porous high-density polyethylene (Medpor) implants to acute and early infection. Arch Otolaryngol Head Neck Surg 1997;123:328–36.

27. Maas CS, Merwin GE, Wilson J, et al. Comparison of biomaterials for facial bone augmentation. Arch Otolaryngol Head Neck Surg 1990;116:551–6.

28. Prendergast M, Schoenrock LD. Malar augmentation. Arch Otolaryngol Head Neck Surg 1989;115:964–9.

29. Jabaley ME, Hoopes JE, Cochran TC. Transoral Silastic augmentation of the malar region. Br J Plast Surg 1974;27:98–102.

30. Rubin JP, Yaremchuk MJ. Complications and toxicities of implantable biomaterials used in facial reconstructive and aesthetic surgery: a comprehensive review of the literature. Plast Reconstr Surg 1997;100(5):1336–53.

Lip Lift

Angela Sturm, MD[a,b,*]

KEYWORDS

- Lip lift • Bullhorn lip lift • Lip augmentation

KEY POINTS

- Lip lift should achieve a feminine, balanced appearance of the lips and face with a small amount of tooth shown with animation.
- Incision placement and tension distribution are key to optimal results.
- Placing the force of the lift on deeper, stable structures creates more natural results with less perceptable incisions.

INTRODUCTION

Facial gender-affirming surgery should never be a consistent "package" of surgeries, but tailored to each person's features, goals, and dysphoria. Each patient's face should be evaluated as a whole and each feature in that context. When looking at another person's face, the observer looks at the eyes first, unless that person is smiling the observer notices the mouth first according to studies with eye movement registrations, making lips important for the recognition of gender.[1]

Generally, masculine lips have a longer distance between the nasal sill and the vermillion border, a shorter vermillion height, and have less teeth showing with animation or with the mouth slightly open. In a study evaluating labio-oral measurements in attractive masculine and feminine faces, the distance between the sill and vermillion was 22 mm in masculine lips and 20 mm in feminine lips.[2] The total lip vermilion height was determined to be 8.4 mm in masculine faces and 8.9 mm in feminine faces.[2] Hoefflin suggests another way to estimate ideal lip measurements in that the distance from the alar base horizontal to the upper lip vermilion should be the same or shorter than the distance from the ocular supratarsal crease to the lower lid lash line.[3]

A lip lift shortens the distance between the nasal sill and vermillion border, everts the vermillion, and provides the feminine and rejuvenating tooth show.[4] Traditional lip lift techniques have been criticized and avoided out of concern for scarring. To avoid visible scarring, surgeons have tried creative incision designs; however, these procedures cause other complications and some authors call into question the aesthetic

[a] Private Practice; [b] Department of Otolaryngology–Head and Neck Surgery, University of Texas Medical Branch, Galveston, TX, USA
* 6750 West Loop South, Suite 1060, Bellaire, TX 77401.
E-mail address: drsturm@drangelasturm.com

Otolaryngol Clin N Am 55 (2022) 835–847
https://doi.org/10.1016/j.otc.2022.04.013
0030-6665/22/© 2022 Elsevier Inc. All rights reserved.

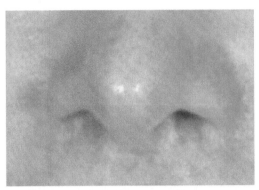

Fig. 1. Flattening of the alar sills, atrophic scarring, and hypopigmentation after advancing lip skin into the nasal sills.

quality of the results.[5] The key to a good outcome is incision design that respects the natural anatomy, placing the tension of the lip deep to the dermis to take tension off of the skin incision, determining the appropriate amount of lift for the patient's anatomy and not violating the orbicularis oris.

History

The upper lip lift has been performed for over 4 decades.[6] In 1971, the "indirect lip lift," which was later called the "bullhorn" lip lift because of the shape of the incision, was introduced by Cardoso and Sperli as a wavy skin excision in the subnasal area.[6,7] Gonzalez-Ulloa described an "L-shaped lip lift" or "philtrum lip lift" excising a bilateral area of skin under the nose and along the ridge of philtrum,[8] similar to the inverted triangular vertical midline excision for patients with a wide philtrum described by Austin in 1986.[4,8,9]

To attempt to minimize the visibility of the subnasal incision, other techniques have reduced the incision length or hidden it in the nostrils. The Greenwald incision has 2 variations that preserve the skin beneath the columella: one resects a strip of orbicularis and is called the "Italian lip lift"[10,11] and the other preserves the orbicularis muscle, which decreases the nasolabial angle and is called the "double duck nasolabial lift."[12] Raphael and colleagues described an endonasal lip lift using skin flaps on the inferior limb of the excision to advance into the nasal sills to hide the subnasal incision. These flaps are anchored to the supraperiosteal tissue along the vestibular floor.[13] However, this technique can lead to the effacement of the nasal sill and either narrowing or widening the nasal sill, changing the nasal proportions.[5] (**Fig. 1**)

Intranasal incisions were used by Echo and colleagues (2011), et al to create a "no scar" lip lift. A full transfixion incision is made, brought along the nasal floor and superiorly as an intercartilaginous incision. Dissection is carried halfway to the vermilion border whereby the orbicularis oris is sutured to the maxillary spine.[14]

Placing the entirety of the tension of the lift on smaller incisions or creating scarring across the nasal sills can lead to the effacement of the nasal base and create an unnatural appearance, which is unfortunately very difficult to correct.[5,8-12] Talei described a modification of the bullhorn technique using a deeper and more extensive release of the upper lip and definitive suspension. With this technique, the dissection is in the sub-superficial muscular aponeurotic system (SMAS) layer, similar to a deep plane facelift. The advantages of this technique are not only placing the tension on the stronger SMAS layer, distributing it across the nasal base, and affixing to the firm pyriform ligament, but keeping the deep sutures in the SMAS layer avoiding suture granulomas or irregular healing from a dermal closure.[5]

Another technique to improve the fullness of the lips is the direct lip lift, also called the vermilion lip lift or "gull wing lip lift" which was first described by Meyer in 1976.[15] This involves removing skin around the vermilion border and advancing the mucosa superiorly and inferiorly to create more fullness. In 1985, Greenwald introduced the corner of the mouth lift and since then various shapes of skin excision were suggested to improve lateral fullness, downturned corners of the mouth, and marionette lines.[4,15–21] In specific patients, this can be useful; however, patient selection is important since, these incisions can be visible, hypertrophic or cause blunting of the vermillion.

Mucosal advancement flaps were also described to increase lip volume without external incisions. A double Y-V transverse flap was first described by Delerm and Elbaz in 1975.[22–24] This results in protrusion of the central vermillion to produce central lip pouting while decreasing the transverse length of the lips. Also, vertical V-to-Y advancements in the intraoral mucosa have been described to evert the lip. In 1991, Aiache described the W-shaped V-Y advancement making 1 or 2 sets of "W" incisions with the bases toward the lip sulcus and tip toward the vermillion mucosal junction.[25] Modifications have been described by Ho, Samiian, Jacono, and Quatela.[26–28] This technique can be used in patients with a short white lip and thin vermillion border. Compared with the indirect lip lift, mucosal advancement has increased the risk of adverse outcomes, prolonged recovery, possible under-correction, and does not change the length of the distance between the nasal sill and vermillion border, so did not gain popularity like the indirect lip lift.[19] (**Fig. 2**)

Lip augmentation with hyaluronic acid is a popular way to improve the lost vermilion volume and height because of the lower patient cost, accessibility, and lack of need for anesthesia. Many patients prefer the temporary nature of hyaluronic acid fillers to "try out" lip augmentation. For many patients, particularly those seeking gender-affirming procedures, a permanent option is preferred. The ideal permanent filler for these patients would be soft, pliable, permanent and lack complications.[29–31] However, no permanent filler exists that is approved for the lips. Many permanent implants are associated with complications, including hardening, shortening, and extrusion in some cases.[32,33] Fat transfer or subaponeurotic system insertion into the lips may require multiple treatments, can have irregularities and resorption is unpredictable.[34,35] In addition, adding volume to the lip does not give an overall rejuvenation of the perioral area because it does not address the lengthening of the white lip or tooth show.[36] Some combine fat augmentation with lip lifting procedures for additional volume.

Evaluation

A thorough history and physical is obtained from all patients. Many patients will present for overall facial evaluation and suggestions, but others will have specific concerns with their lips. Patients most often present with excess white lip length, drooping upper lip, loss of red lip, over-filled lips, filler complications, postsurgical changes in the lips, poorly defined or thin upper lip, asymmetry, and loss of tooth show with animation, creating an aged or masculine appearance. Specifically, tooth show is associated with femininity and sensuality.[5] As the lip lengthens the function is diminished and the definition of the Cupid's bow is lost over time. Asymmetries of the central upper lip and Cupid's bow can also be addressed with the lip lift.

In patients who have had filler placed on their lips, a detailed history should be undertaken to determine the type of filler and if this is reversible. Negative effects of permanent fillers such as silicone, fat, and polymers such as polymethylmethacrylate

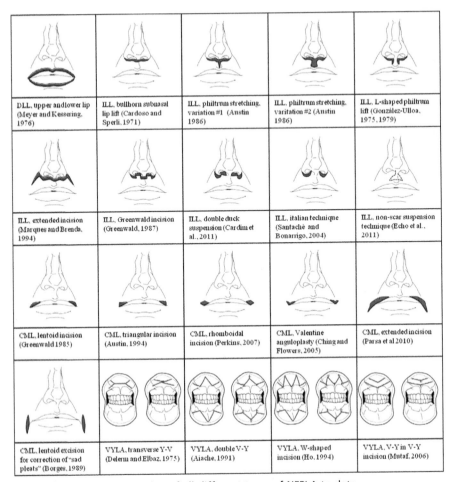

Fig. 2. Schematic representation of all different types of NFPLA to date.

(PMMA) can cause permanent damage due to expansion, thickening, and effacement, as well as inhibiting function. Temporary fillers such as hyaluronic acid dermal fillers have complications such as migration above the vermillion border, limitation in movement, irregularities, and vascular complications.[5] In particular, Talei describes more persistence and migration with Juvederm XC, which the author has seen, as well.[5] Migrated filler is notably found in the 10 mm segment superior to the vermillion border up to years after the injection. If a hyaluronic acid filler is present, it is advisable to dissolve before the lip lift for optimal results and reduction in postoperative inflammation.[5] A history of surgical procedures such as rhinoplasty or orthognathic surgery can cause the lengthening of the upper lip. Maneuvers to deproject the tip, full transfixion incisions, or dissection around the nasal base can cause elongation of the lip and hypomobility immediately following surgery.[5]

A physical examination and facial analysis using the vertical fifths and horizontal thirds is essential to evaluate the upper lip in the context of the entire face. An attractive mouth has a short "prolabium" of the upper lip, prominent and defined "philtrum" and Cupid's bow, more defined vermillion in the central part of the lips, lower lip that is slightly fuller than the upper lip, and visible upper incisors with partially closed mouth.

A masculine lip has a longer upper lip, less red lip volume, less tooth show, and disappearance of the Cupid's bow.[11]

Ideal candidates are those whom the effect of the lip lift would create facial balance, enhance the perioral complex including the patient's dentition and not create and exaggerated appearance.[5] An ideal tooth show with the mouth gently opened for patients with normal occlusion can be approximately 3 mm.[7] However, the facial shape, dentition, occlusion and overall facial appearance will guide the surgical decision making. Patients with a significant dental overjet, malocclusion, gaunt appearance, suboptimal dentition, maxillary-mandibular imbalance, or those for whom a fuller lip would look disproportionate may not be ideal candidates or may be considered for a conservative lift and referral to a dental colleague.[5] Patients with downturn of the corners of the mouth can be candidates for a corner mouth lift.[4,17–19]

Surgical Techniques

The sub-nasal incision remains the standard approach to lip lifting. With both the Bullhorn and modified lip lift, the landmarks of mid-columella, lateral columella, center of right nostril sill, center of right ala, center of left nostril sill, and center of left ala are marked and lines are drawn from these landmarks to the white roll to make the lift more precise and symmetric. The superior incision is placed in or 1 mm inferior to the alar-facial crease on each side not invading the sill. Multiple authors advocate

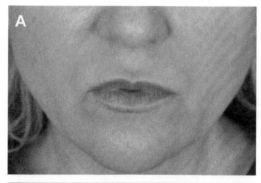

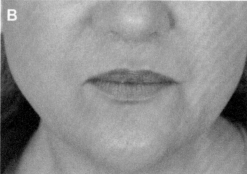

Fig. 3. The modified lip lift technique was used to place the incision in the alar facial crease and the deep sutures in the superficial aponeurotic muscular system so that the incision heals such that it is nearly imperceptible over time. By adjusting the lift on each side, asymmetries of the vermillion were improved, while creating a more feminine, relaxed, sensual, and balanced lip.

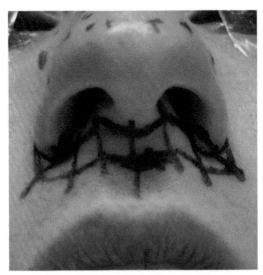

Fig. 4. The incision is placed in or 1mm inferior to the alar facial crease preserving the sill. The incision starts laterally at but not past the well-demarcated alar crease, medially in or 1mm inferior to the alar facial crease crurving medially to the superior edge of the philtral column where it creates a peak, then curves along the inferior aspect of the columella on each side. The landmarks of the mid-columella, superior edge of philtral column or lateral columella if the philtral column is not defined, mid sill and mid-ala are marked. In this patient, the inferior limb is placed at the horizontal crease created while smiling, which is approximately 4mm inferior to the alar-facial crease. The landmarks are marked at 4mm with a caliper and connected mirroring the superior limb.

not violating the nostril sill because the scar is well-hidden in the nostril crease below the sill and is usually imperceptible.[4,5] (**Fig. 3**) Laterally the incision goes to but not past the well-demarcated alar crease to reduce visibility. The incision is carried medially creating a peak at the superior edge of the philtral, then it curves along the inferior aspect of the columella (**Fig. 4**).

In the bullhorn technique, the inferior limb is then drawn with the widest portion of the excision beneath the ala and a narrower excision centrally to create a lift more laterally and a more superior medial lift.[7] The location of the inferior limb is determined by the amount of skin excision and lift is planned. Frequently patients will have a horizontal crease that forms with smiling that creates a natural position for the lower limb. If that limb doesn't exist or a more objective measurement is preferred, the amount of skin excision for a conservative lip lift is 3–5 mm, an average lift is 5–7 mm and an aggressive excision is 7 to 9 mm.[5] Intentional asymmetric resection can address asymmetries in the vermillion border.

In addition, the amount of desired tooth show is also an excellent way to decide the amount of skin excision. The average amount of upper tooth shown at age 25 is 3.5 mm. By the age of 45, the average person does not have tooth show with the lips slightly parted.[9] Therefore, restoring the 3 mm of tooth show gives a feminine, soft, rejuvenated appearance to the face.[7] For most patients, the minimum amount of remaining lip from nostril sill to the Cupid's bow is 11 mm and leaving less than 10 mm is not recommended because it can look too short regardless of incisor show.[4]

A lip lift can be performed under local anesthesia or under general anesthesia when combined with other feminization procedures. Oral anxiolysis is recommended because of the discomfort associated with the local anesthetic. The incision is made perpendicular to the skin down to the junction of the fat and muscle. The skin and subcutaneous layer are removed leaving a layer of fat over the orbicularis, ensuring the vasculature deep to the SMAS, such as the inferior alar arteries remain intact.[5]

The original description of the Bullhorn lip lift described a 3 mm inferior skin flap to ensure eversion of the dermis with closure.[7,36] However, the author prefers the modified upper lip lift, in which dissection is then carried in the plane inferior to the SMAS plane release the SMAS from the orbicularis oris. The SMAS is a discrete, strong tissue layer just deep into the reticular dermis.[37] The dissection is carried far enough inferiorly and laterally to allow a minimal tension closure. This is usually approximately half-way down the central philtrum and to the nasolabial folds bilaterally. The lift should be more laterally than centrally to avoid an unnatural or "hare lip" appearance. Dissection to the vermillion is not advised because it risks the effacement of the cupid's bow. Staying sub-SMAS allows the surgeon to avoid bleeding or damage to the mimetic muscles. Careful hemostasis is achieved. The SMAS on the labial flap is then suspended to a firm structure with 5 to 0 PDS sutures to prevent the widening of the incision and poor scarring that is seen with a dermal closure alone.[5] The pyriform ligament serves as a perfectly stable structure that can be sutured with deep absorbable sutures.[37] The pyriform ligament is preferred to maxillary periosteum because anchoring the suture to the periosteum can create an exaggeration of the tacking of the labial flap that is difficult to repair. Suturing to the SMAS allows the dermal edges to be brought together to allow tension-free approximation with nonabsorbable interrupted sutures. Meticulous closure with either 6 to 0 nylon or Prolene interrupted and mattress sutures is imperative to make the incision as imperceptible as possible.[5]

Patient expectations for healing should be set preoperatively. Postoperatively, the patient can expect swelling at the incision, but in the upper lip, as well. As with most surgeries, the full healing process may be a year, but the recovery time is approximately 3 months before the result can start to be appreciated. The incision may require injections of 5-fluorouracil or Kenalog or resurfacing for optimal results.[5]

Lip lifts are frequently performed in conjunction with other procedures to feminize the face, which often includes rhinoplasty. Some plastic surgeons have debated the safety of performing open rhinoplasty with a transcolumellar incision and a lip lift with a separate sub-nasal incision leaving an island of columellar skin for fear of skin necrosis or excessive scarring.[38] However, there is no data on the literature to support this theory and there are numerous studies demonstrating the robust blood supply of the columella.[39–42] In addition, Insalaco and Speigel showed otherwise in a retrospective review of 105 cases of simultaneous lip-lift and rhinoplasty using 2 columellar incisions and in some cases alar base reductions, as well, there were no incidences of columellar deformity, necrosis or other healing problems.[43] (**Fig. 5**)

Sub-nasal lip lifts can be performed in conjunction with lateral or corner lip lifts in patients with downturned corners of the lips that create unhappy or harsh appearances. In these patients, a corner lip lift creates a more serene, pleasant, balanced appearance.[4] A number of shapes for excision have been proposed, including a simple ellipse excision of skin which is performed at the lateral upper lip margin to advance the vermillion superiorly. The incision is created at the vermillion border and can be wrapped around the vermilion edge to avoid irregularities or depression at the incision.[16,18,19] The incision can be carried medially up to but not violating the Cupid's bow.[4]

Complications/Concerns

The perioral area is visible, dynamic, and unforgiving of irregularities and scarring, so incision design is critical. Attempts have been made to shorten the incision or hide it in

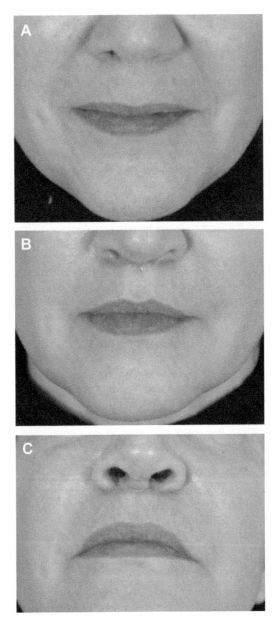

Fig. 5. Before (*A*) and after (*B*) early results after suture removal for a patient who underwent revision rhinoplasty with a mid-columellar incision and lip lift with a subnasal incision. The blood supply to the columella is strong and tolerates both incisions well (*C*).

the nasal sills. However, shortening the incision can lead to the inability to redistribute the skin evenly, and lift only the central lip only creating a "hare lip" appearance or downturn of the upper lip. Furthermore, a shortened scar can place increased tension on the smaller incisions creating poor healing and effacement of the alar base. This effacement can become more prominent in cases whereby sill tissue is removed, and lip skin is advanced into the nostrils. With these techniques, the tension of the lift is also placed across the sills creating a further flattening (**Fig. 6**). Unfortunately, once the sill tissue is removed and scarring occurs, this cannot be replaced or repaired.[5] The study by Raphael and colleagues describes complications of alar distortion (12%), sill widening (9%) sill deformation (13%), and change in nostril shape.[13] Even this study discussed improvement but not the elimination of these complications with their improved understanding of nasal anatomy with time and preserving subdermal sill anatomy.[13] Therefore, optimal incision design is below the natural curves of the nasal base to the lateral natural curve of the ala. Other complications include hypertrophic scarring, under correction, infection, suture abscess, long-standing edema for up to 3 months, and unraveled sutures.[9,11,12,14,36,44]

Using the intranasal incisions described by Echo, and colleagues to create a "no scar" lip lift can cause scarring at the intercartilaginous incisions causing changes in nasal shape, nasal tip change from advancing columellar skin superiorly, and tip deprojection from the full transfixion incision.[14] Attempts to excise, suspend or plicate the orbicularis oris muscle cause trauma to a dynamic and sensitive muscle causing hypokinesis of the lip, which can change the smile and reduce tooth show.[5,11] Hypokinesis and paresthesias were exhibited by most of the patients in the study by Echo, and colleagues, in which suspension of the orbicularis oris was described.[14] In the study by Talei for which the deep sutures were placed in the orbicularis, but the SMAS, there were no cases of hypokinesis.[5] Fibrosis caused by suturing the orbicularis oris can also pull the alar base inferiorly creating a widening of the incision and relative increased the tip rotation of the nose.[5,11]

The risk of hematoma only exists in the modified lip lift whereby a labial flap is created. The study by Talei had 2 patients out of 823 with minor hematomas.[5] In the other descriptions of the bullhorn, indirect or subnasal lip lift, a potential space is not created; therefore, the risk of hematoma is eliminated. However, these techniques have an increased risk of tension due to insufficient tissue dissection of the flaps creating widened or hypertrophic scarring.[5] In the study by Holden, and colleagues, the subnasal lip lift was performed with skin excision and dermal closure. Of these patients, 20% required dermabrasion to the incision.[36] In the systematic review by Morogas of subnasal lip lifts without labial flaps, only 22.3% of people were satisfied with the procedure in the first 6 months without makeup. After 1 year, patient satisfaction was over 80% in all groups, demonstrating that the procedure does have an extended recovery time and patients' expectations should be set preoperatively.[45]

Direct lip lifts at the vermillion border cause a visible scar, hypertrophic scarring, under-correction, asymmetry, infection, and flattening of the vermillion border requiring camouflage with makeup.[9,36,46,47] In the systematic review by Moragas, 5 of the 6 articles about direct lip lift talk about the utility of lipstick after surgery, leading the author to that a completely natural look after this procedure without makeup is unlikely.[45] In the event that a lateral lip lift is required for the patient, this should not be carried across the Cupid's bow to prevent this flattening.[5]

The V-Y lip advancements were associated with significant edema in 100% of the patients in the study by Aiache and 9.4% were debilitating for 3 weeks, 79% led to difficulty eating or articulating words and inability to purse one's lips or use straws, asymmetry with posterior revision in 25%, under-correction, overcorrection, paresthesias, hypoesthesia, dehiscence of mucosal advancement and dryness of lips in 75% of patients.[25–27,47,48]

DISCUSSION

Lip lifting adds a softening and feminizing of the entire face that is valuable in facial gender-affirming surgery. Augmentation of the lips with soft tissue filler or fat can

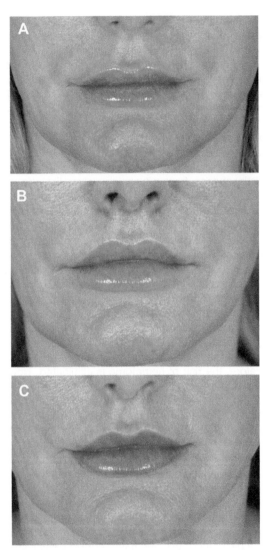

Fig. 6. Even when subdermal sill anatomy is respected, but the incision is placed across it, the sill architecture frequently flattens with healing forces and tension in that area. The (*A*) before shows a long distance between the sill and vermillion and less vermillion fullness. Early in the healing process (*B*) the sill architecture is maintained, the distance between the sill and vermillion is improved, as is the fullness. After a year, (*C*) the lip fullness and position are improved, but the incision has some atrophy.

increase the fullness but does not address the distance between the nasal sill and vermillion and improve tooth show, unlike the lip lift. Often patients become over-filled trying to achieve the feminine, youthful lip with the wrong tool. Mucosal advancements provide volume, but tend to have significant prolonged swelling, paresthesias, and hypokinesis making these procedures less than ideal. Direct lip lifts cause scarring at the vermillion border which can be visible, hypertrophic, or blunt the vermillion border. Lateral lip lifts have some limited utility in specific patients with downturned corners of the mouth.

Concerns and opposition to performing the lip lift are always centered around the visibility of the incision. Given the central location and mobility of the perioral area, this does pose issues with camouflaging incisions and healing. The evolution of the lip lift involved variations in hiding the incision and supporting the lift. The complexity of the lip lift does not lie in the difficulty of the surgical technique, but in the finesse of the details and preventing of complications. Higher rates of complications were found with lifts with deep closure in the dermis and incisions that violate the nasal sill.[5,13,14,36] Limited incisions may create an uneven or unnatural lift while placing the tension on less surface area, which can efface the nasal base and cause widened incisions. An incision that spans from the lateral nasal ala, inferior to the sill, and across the inferior columella does not violate the sill will avoid volume loss and scarring in the sill and distributes the force of the lift in broader distribution. Placing the force of the lift on the SMAS to the stable pyriform ligament further reduces the force on the incision and obviates the need for sutures in the dermis that can cause granulomas and irregular healing.[5]

SUMMARY

A long distance between the nasal sill and vermillion, thin upper lip, and lack of tooth show with animation and slight opening of the mouth can create a masculine appearance to the lower third of the face and appearance as a whole. Care should be taken to create a natural, balanced lip shape and make the incision as imperceptible as possible. Taking the tension off the skin closure and maintaining native anatomy are keys to achieving these results.

CLINICS CARE POINTS

- Traditionally, an attractive mouth has a short "prolabium" of the upper lip, prominent and defined "philtrum" and Cupid's bow. more defined vermillion in the central part of the lips, lower lip that is slightly fuller than the upper lip, and visible upper incisors with a partially closed mouth.

- The incision has been described in various ways, but the traditional bullhorn is an ellipse from the lateral aspect of the alar crease to the landmarks of mid-sill, lateral columella to the mid-columella bilaterally in the alar-facial crease with the inferior limb placement decided by the amount of lift desired.

- Incisions across the nasal sill can lead to nasal base effacement and poor scarring.

- Generally, the amount of skin excision for a conservative lip lift is 3–5 mm, an average lift is 5–7 mm and an aggressive excision is 7 to 9 mm.

- The desired tooth show can be used to determine the amount of skin excision and the average tooth show to achieve a natural, feminine appearance is approximately 3 mm.

- For most patients, the minimum amount of remaining lip from nostril sill to the Cupid's bow is 11 mm and leaving less than 10 mm is not recommended.

- The tension of the lift should not be on the dermis or orbicularis oris, but on the submucosal aponeurotic system to avoid poor scarring and hypomobility.

DISCLOSURE

Dr A. Sturm is a Luminary for Lutronic USA for devices unrelated to this content. The author has no conflicts of interest relevant to the content of this article.

REFERENCES

1. Yarbus AL. Eye Movements during examination of complex objects. Biofizika 1961;6:207–e227.
2. Farkas LG. Anthropometry of the attractive North American caucasian face. In: Anthropometry of the head and face13, 2nd edition. New York: Raven Press; 1994. p. 159–68.
3. Hoefflin SM. The labial ledge. Aesthet Surg J 2002;22:177–80.
4. Weston GW, Poindexter BD, Sigal RK, et al. Lifting lips: 28 years of experience using the direct excision approach to rejuvenating the aging mouth. Aesthet Surg J 2009;29:83–6.
5. Talei B. The Modified upper lip lift advanced approach with deep-plane release and secure suspension: 823-patient series. Facial Plast Surg Clin North Am 2019;27:385–98.
6. Cardoso AD, Sperli AE. Rhytidoplasty of the upper lip. transactions of the fifth international congress of plastic and reconstructive surgery. Sydney (Australia): Butterworth-Heinemann; 1971. p. 1127–9.
7. Ramirez OM, Khan AS, Robertson KM. The upper lip lift using the "bull's horn" approach. J Drugs Dermatol 2003;3:305–8.
8. Gonzalez-Ulloa M. The aging upper lip. Ann Plast Surg 1979;2(4):299–303.
9. Austin HW. The lip lift. Plast Reconstr Surg 1986;77:990–4.
10. Greenwald AE. The lip lift. Plast Reconstr Surg 1987;79(1):147.
11. Santanchè P, Bonarrigo C. Lifting of the upper lip: personal technique. Plast Reconstr Surg 2004;113(6):1828–35. Techniques in Cosmetic Surgery. 2003; revised August 19, 2003.
12. Cardim VLN, Dos Santos A, Locas R, et al. Double Duck nasolabial lifting. Rev Bras Cir 2011;26:466–71.
13. Raphael P, Harris R, Harris SW. The endonasal lip lift: personal technique. Aesthet Surg J 2014;34(3):457–68.
14. Echo A, Momoh AO, Yuksel E. The no-scar lip-lift: upper lip suspension Technique. Aesth Plast Surg 2011;35:617–23.
15. Meyer R, Kesserling UK. Aesthetic surgery in the perioral region. Aesthetic Plast Surg 1976;1:619.
16. Greenwald A. The lip lift: cheiloplexy for cheiloptosis. Am J Cos Surg 1985;2(16).
17. Austin HW. Rejuvenating the aging mouth. Semin Plast Surg 1994;8:27–e56.
18. Poindexter BD, Sigal RK, Austin HW, et al. Surgical treatment of the aging mouth. Semin Plast Surg 2003;17:199–208.
19. Perkins SW. The corner of the mouth lift and management of the oral commissure grooves. Facial Plast Surg Clin North Am 2007;15:471–6.
20. Parsa FD, Parsa NN, Murariu D. Surgical correction of the frowning mouth. Plast Reconstr Surg 2010;125:667–76.
21. Borges AF. Sad pleats. Ann Plast Surg 1989;22:74–5.
22. Delerm A, Elbaz JA. Chelioplastie des levres minces. propostion d'une technique. Am Chir Plast 1975;20:243–9.
23. Lassus C. Thickening the thin lips. Plast Reconstr Surg 1981;68:950–e952.
24. Lassus C. Surgical vermillion augmentation: different possibilities. Aesthetic Plast Surg 1992;16:123–e127.
25. Aiache AE. Augmentation cheiloplasty. Plast Reconstr Surg 1991;88:222–e226.
26. Ho LCY. Augmentation cheiloplasty. Br J Plast Surg 1994;47:257–e262.
27. Samiian MR. Lip augmentation for correction of thin lips. Plast Reconstr Surg 1993;911:162–e166.

28. Jacono AA, Quatela VC. Quantitative analysis of lip appearance after VeY lip augmentation. Arch Facial Plast Surg 2004;6:172–e177.
29. Sclafani AP, Romo T III, Jacono AA. Rejuvenation of the aging lip with an injectable acellular dermal graft (Cymetra). Arch Facial Plast Surg 2002;4(4):252–7.
30. Tzikas TL. Evaluation of the radiance FN soft tissue filler for facial soft tissue augmentation. Arch Facial Plast Surg 2004;6(4):234–9.
31. Cox SE. Who is still using expanded polytetrafluoroethylene? Dermatol Surg 2005;31(11, pt 2):1613–5.
32. Rubin JP, Yaremchuk MJ. Complications and toxicities of implantable biomaterials used in facial reconstructive and aesthetic surgery: a comprehensive review of the literature. Plast Reconstr Surg 1997;100(5):1336–53.
33. Recupero WD, McCollough EG. Comparison of lip enhancement using autologous superficial musculoaponeurotic system tissue and postauricular fascia in conjunction with lip advancement. Arch Facial Plast Surg 2010;12(5):342–8.
34. Gatti JE. Permanent lip augmentation with serial fat grafting. Ann Plast Surg 1999; 42(4):376–80.
35. Boahene KDO, Orten SS, Hilger PA. Facial analysis of the rhinoplasty patient. In: Papel ID, editor. Facial and reconstructive surgery. 3rd edtion. New York: Thieme Medical Publishers Inc; 2009. p. 477–8.
36. Holden PK, Sufyan AS, Perkins SW. Long-term analysis of surgical correction of the senile upper lip. Arch Facial Plast Surg 2011;13(5):332–6.
37. Rohrich RJ, Hoxworth RE, Thornton JF, et al. The pyriform ligament. Plast Reconstr Surg 2008;121(1):277–81.
38. Nahai F. The art of aesthetic surgery: principles and techniques. 2nd edition. St Louis (MO): Quality Medical Publishing; 2011. p. 1796–821.
39. Rohrich RJ, Gunter JP, Friedman RM. Nasal tip blood supply: an anatomic study validating the safety of the transcolumellar incision in rhinoplasty. Plast Reconstr Surg 1995;95(5):795–9.
40. Toriumi DM, Mueller RA, Grosch T, et al. Vascular anatomy of the nose and the external rhinoplasty approach. Arch Otolaryngol Head Neck Surg 1996;122(1): 24–34.
41. Bafaqeeh SA, Al-Qattan MM. Simultaneous open rhinoplasty and alar base excision: is there a problem with the blood supply of the nasal tip and columellar skin? Plast Reconstr Surg 2000;105(1):344–7.
42. Tellioğlu AT, Vargel I, Cavuşoğlu T, et al. Simultaneous open rhinoplasty and alar base excision for secondary cases. Aesthetic Plast Surg 2005;29(3):151–5.
43. Insalaco L, Spiegel JH. Safety of simultaneous lip-lift and open rhinoplasty. JAMA Facial Plast Surg 2017;19(2):160–1.
44. Marques A, Brenda E. Lifting of the upper lip using a single extensive incision. Br J Plast Surg 1994;47(1):50–3.
45. Moragas JSM, Vercruysse HJ, Mommaerts MY. Non-filling" procedures for lip augmentation: a systematic review of contemporary techniques and their outcomes. J Craniomaxillofac Surg 2014;42:943–52.
46. Fanous N. Correction of thin lips: "Lip lift. Plast Reconstr Surg 1984;74:33.
47. Haworth RD. Customizing perioral enhancement to obtain ideal lip aesthetids: combining both lip voluming and reshaping procedures by means of an algorithmic approach. Plast Reconstr Surg 2004;113:2182–92.
48. Mutaf M. V-Y in V-Y procedure: new technique for augmentation and protrusion of the upper lip. Ann Plast Surg 2006;56:605–8.

3D Sliding Genioplasty and Its Role in Facial Feminization Surgery

Cvetan Taskov, MD

KEYWORDS

- 3D sliding genioplasty • T genioplasty • Facial feminization surgery
- Narrowing sliding genioplasty • Facial feminization • Facial harmonization
- Chin reduction

KEY POINTS

- In the hands of an expereienced surgeon, is this procedure a very safe surgery with prdictable results.
- By means of 3D sliding genioplasty the size, form, height, position, and proportions of the chin in all dimensions can be altered.
- The 3D sliding genioplasty is a very effective and precise feminizing procedure.

The chin is the main element of the lower third of the face. It influences the appearance and aesthetics of the face significantly.[1] The male chin is wide and angular, often with lateral prominences. This leads to the broad and dominant appearance of the chin and of the lower third of the face in men. In women, the chin is rather tapered and oval.

Other issues such as width, height, length, and position of the chin can also affect its appearance.

The German surgeon Hofer[2] was the first person who reportedly (1942) proposed a horizontal osteotomy with the advancement of the lower fragment for the treatment of microgenia. Gillies wrote in the 1950s in "The principles and art of plastic surgery" by Gillies and Millard,[3] about the "jumping" genioplasty to shorten or advance the lower border of the chin. Since the introduction of the osseous genioplasty by Trauner and Obwegeser in 1957,[4] genioplasty has become very popular and highly established for the treatment of various conditions. With this procedure, we can alter the size, form, height, position, and proportions of the chin in all dimensions and that's why we call it 3D sliding genioplasty.[5]

SURGICAL PROCEDURE

All surgeries are performed under general anesthesia using orotracheal intubation and are performed intraorally. The incision is made after infiltration of 1% Xylocaine and 1:100,000 Epinephrine. The infiltration is made submucosal along the incision line and subperiosteal

Praxis für Plastische und Ästhetische Chirurgie Erding, Angermair-Haus, 3. Obergeschoß, Franz-Brombach-Str. 11-13, Erding 85435, Germany
E-mail address: praxis@dr-taskov.de

Otolaryngol Clin N Am 55 (2022) 849–858
https://doi.org/10.1016/j.otc.2022.04.008
0030-6665/22/© 2022 Elsevier Inc. All rights reserved.

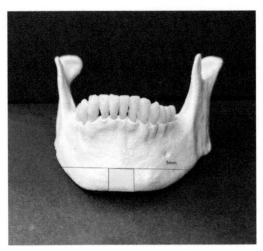

Fig. 1. Frontal illustration of a narrowing sliding genioplasty.

in the area of dissection. A labial incision is made 1 cm distal to the labial sulcus between the 2 canines. If additional procedures, like V-line surgery, mandible angle resection,[6,7] or lateral cortex ostectomy are needed, we perform 2 additional incisions along the sulcus from the canine to the anterior edge of the ascending ramus of the mandible.

The dissection is done subperiosteal. Care should be taken not to deglove the inferior border of the mandible completely and not injure the mental nerves. Complete degloving of the bone will lead to the malperfusion of the bone segments.

According to the presurgical planning, the osteotomy lines are marked on the chin by means of scoring with the reciprocating saw.

With the 3D sliding genioplasty, it is possible to alter the width, height, length, and position of the chin in all directions. This procedure is able to narrow, advance/reduce, and shorten/lengthen the chin.

To achieve narrowing of the chin, a horizontal osteotomy should be done at least 5 mm below the mental foramen (**Figs. 1** and **2**). Two parallel vertical osteotomies

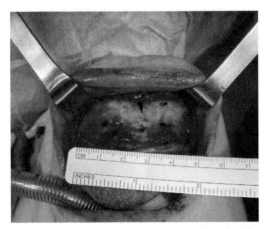

Fig. 2. Photographs of a narrowing sliding genioplasty combined with a mandibular lateral cortex ostectomy procedure. Osteotomy planning.

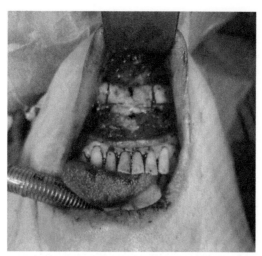

Fig. 3. Photographs of a narrowing sliding genioplasty combined with a mandibular lateral cortex ostectomy procedure. Horizontal osteotomy and 2 vertical osteotomies are performed.

are done in the central portion of chin.[8] The distance between the 2 vertical osteotomies is according to the pre-surgical planning and determines the narrowing of the chin. Segment resection of up to 2 cm is possible. All osteotomies are performed by means of a reciprocating saw. The central segment is then dissected and removed. The lose distal segments are now approximated and fixed with a titanium plate and screws. The lose musculature will be adapted and multi-point fixed with 2/0 Polyglactin (Vicryl), so that no hollow space is left and chin ptosis can be prevented.

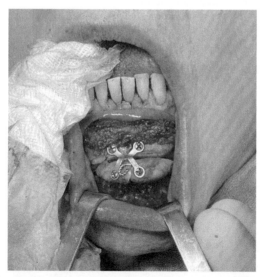

Fig. 4. Photographs of a narrowing sliding genioplasty combined with a mandibular lateral cortex ostectomy procedure. After removal of the central segment, the 2 lateral segments are approximated medially and fixed with a titanium stairstep miniplate.

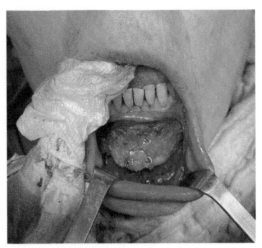

Fig. 5. Photographs of a narrowing sliding genioplasty combined with a mandibular lateral cortex ostectomy procedure. Spaces between the bone segments are filled with bone paste.

To achieve forward/backward sliding or advancement/reduction of the chin, it is necessary to use a pre-bent "stairstep" titanium plate (see **Fig. 2**; **Figs. 3–5**). After removing the central segment, the 2 sides are advanced or reduced as they are brought together. These plates have fixed advancement of 2 to 10 mm and can be used in both directions flipped around-forward and backward. The plates are fixed with titanium screws.

To achieve shortening of the chin, a second parallel horizontal osteotomy is needed (**Figs. 6–10**). The distance between the 2 horizontal lines determines the overall chin shortening. The horizontal segment is dissected and removed. The distal segment is then fixed with titanium plate and screws.

As an alternative to this technique, an "A" shaped osteotomy is also possible (**Fig. 11**). With this procedure, shortening and narrowing of the chin can also simultaneously be achieved.

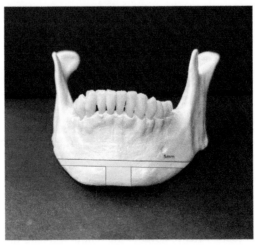

Fig. 6. 3D sliding genioplasty osteotomy planning.

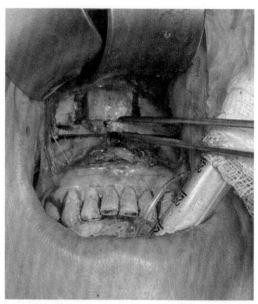

Fig. 7. 3D sliding genioplasty. After performing the 2 vertical osteotomies, 2 parallel horizontal osteotomies are completed.

After the 3D sliding genioplasty is completed, the mandible is inspected and step-off deformities of the chin-mandible junction as well as sharp margins are detected and resected. If additional procedures, such as mini V-line, V-line surgery, or lateral cortex ostectomy,[9] are planned, they will include the step-off deformity. All osteotomies are

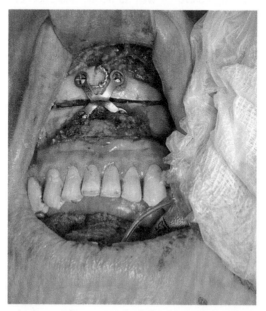

Fig. 8. 3D sliding genioplasty. After removal of the horizontal and central segment, the 2 lateral segments are approximated medially and fixed with a titanium stairstep miniplate.

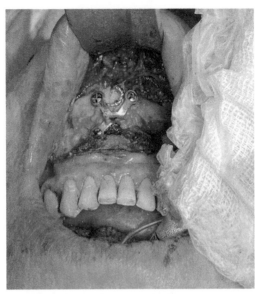

Fig. 9. 3D sliding genioplasty. Spaces between the bone segments are filled with bone paste.

performed with a reciprocating saw. At the end of the procedure, the sharp margins are reduced and smoothed with a burr or a bone file to create the natural shape of the lower margin of the mandible.

The 3D sliding genioplasty has the major advantage of being a very precise and feminizing procedure. Aggressive as well as subtle alteration of size, height, form, and position of the chin is possible. In comparison a shaving procedure alone will

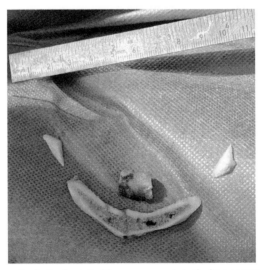

Fig. 10. 3D sliding genioplasty. Resected bone segments including correction of the step-off deformity.

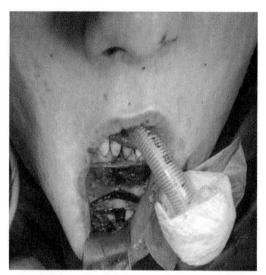

Fig. 11. "A" shaped osteotomy.

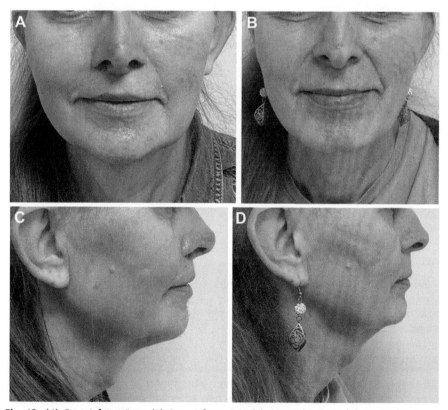

Fig. 12. (*A*) Case 1 front Post. (*B*) Case 1 front Pre. (*C*) Case 1 lat Post. (*D*) Case 1 lat Pre.

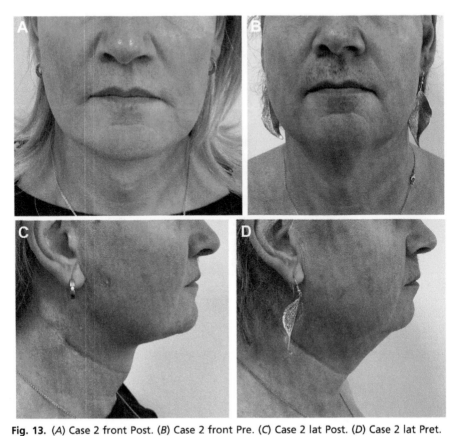

Fig. 13. (*A*) Case 2 front Post. (*B*) Case 2 front Pre. (*C*) Case 2 lat Post. (*D*) Case 2 lat Pret.

affect the size and form of the chin but not its position. Aggressive Shaving may lead to receding chin or chin ptosis.

CASE STUDY 1

A 60-year-old transgender female patient has undergone a 3D sliding genioplasty with 20 mm refinement and 2 mm advancement. In addition, a mandible angle resection, lateral cortex ostectomy lip lift, and a feminizing rhinoplasty were performed (**Fig. 12**).

CASE STUDY 2

A 63-year-old transgender female patient has undergone a 3D sliding genioplasty with 10 mm refinement and 6 mm advancement. A lateral cortex ostectomy, mandible angle resection, lip lift, neck liposuction, and a deep plane facelift have been performed in addition (**Fig. 13**).

CASE STUDY 3

A 25-year-old transgender female patient has undergone a 3D sliding genioplasty with 10 mm refinement, 4 mm shortening and 6 mm advancement. A lateral cortex ostectomy, mandible angle resection has been performed in addition (**Fig. 14**).

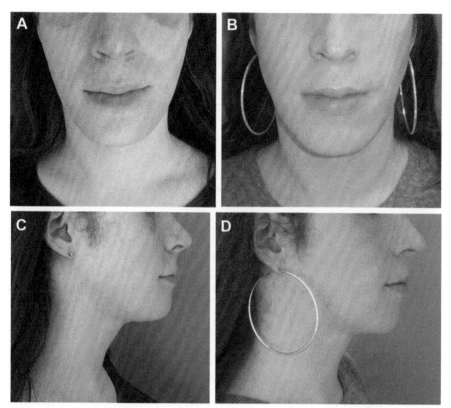

Fig. 14. (*A*) Case 3 front Post. (*B*) Case 3front Pre. (*C*) Case 3 lat Post. (*D*) Case 3 lat Pre.

COMPLICATIONS AND MANAGEMENT
Neurosensory deficiency

Neurosensory deficiency of the lower lip, after sliding genioplasty, is a common complication. Normally this is a temporary condition. To avoid this complication, we recommend careful dissection around the mental foramen without extensive exposure to the mental nerves. In cases with extensive dissection, as in V line surgery, care should be taken not to overextend or even rupture the nerves. In case of a nerve rupture, we recommend immediate microsurgical coaptation with 10/0 Polyamide, otherwise it will result in a permanent sensory loss in this area.

Step-off deformities

Step-off deformities of the chin-mandible junction exceeding 3-4 mm as well as sharp margins or border irregularities should be detected and resected or shaved.

Chin ptosis

In major reduction 3D sliding genioplasty if the soft tissue is not carefully reattached, in older patients with skin excess chin ptosis may occur. To avoid chin ptosis we recommend careful multipoint reattachment of the muscles with 2/0 Polyglactin.

Pseudarthrosis

Maljunction of the dissected bone segments may also appear. To avoid this condition, a careful dissection and incision of the bony fragments is recommended. It is essential to save the muscles attachments in this way is good perfusion of the segments is ensured. In addition, we add bone paste to the segment gaps.

The 3D sliding genioplasty is a very effective and precise feminizing procedure. It enables the surgeon to modify the size, form, height, and position of the chin in all dimensions.[10] The chin is one of the keystone areas of the face. Even subtle alteration of the height, width, or position of the chin can make a tremendous difference in the appearance and aesthetics of the face of a transgender female.

REFERENCES

1. Rosen HM. Aesthetic guidelines in genioplasty: The role of facial disproportion. Plast Reconstr Surg 1995;95:463–9.
2. Hofer O. Die operative Behandlung der alveolaren Retraktiondes Unterkiefers und ihre Anwendungsmöglichkeit für Prognathie und Mikrogenie. Dtsch Z Mund Kieferheilkunde 1942;9:130.
3. Gillies H, Millard D Jr. The principles and art of plastic surgery. Boston: Little Brown & Co; 1975.
4. Trauner R, Obwegeser H. Surgical correction of mandibular prognathism and retrognathism with consideration of genioplasty. Oral Surg 1957;10:677.
5. Hwang K. Importance of the chin in lower facial contour: Narrowing genioplasty to achieve a feminine and slim lower face. Plast Reconstr Surg 2013;132:877e–8e.
6. Park S, Noh JH. Importance of the chin in lower facial contour: narrowing genioplasty to achieve a feminine and slim lower face. Plast Reconstr Surg 2008;122: 261–8.
7. Lee TS, Kim HY, Kim T, et al. Importance of the cnin in achieving a feminine lower face: narrowing the chin by the "mini V-line" surgery. J Craniofac Surg 2014;25: 2180–3.
8. Lee TS, Kim HY, Kim TH, et al. Contouring of the lower face by a novel method of narrowing and lengthening genioplasty. Plast Reconstr Surg 2014;133:274e–82e.
9. Li J, Hsu Y, Khadka A, et al. Contouring of a square jaw on a short face by narrowing and sliding genioplasty combined with mandibular outer cortex ostectomy in Orientals. Plast Reconstr Surg 2011;127:2083–92.
10. Grime PD, Blenkinsopp PT. Horizontal-T genioplasty (a modified technique for the broad or asymmetrical chin). Br J Oral Maxillofac Surg 1990;28:215–21.

Jaw Reduction Surgery

Harrison H. Lee, MD, DMD[a,b,*], Mansher Singh, MD[a]

KEYWORDS

- Facial feminization surgery • Jaw reduction surgery • Transgender patients
- Genioplasty

KEY POINTS

- There is a significant difference in male and female facial features, which can be surgically altered during facial feminization surgery (FFS).
- Jaw reduction surgery is a critical component of FFS.
- We discuss our techniques and pearls of jaw reduction surgery based on our experience of more than 3000 patients.

INTRODUCTION: HISTORY OF JAW CONTOURING

Craniofacial surgery, which includes operating on facial bones, was developed by pioneers in plastic surgery such as Dr Paul Tessier and others around the 1940s. It was not until a few decades later that esthetic surgical correction of facial bones developed as a subspecialty within plastic surgery.[1] However, facial bone contouring surgery really came of age with the introduction and popularization of mandible reduction by Baek.[2] In Asian countries, facial bone surgery and chin and jaw contouring esthetic procedures gathered steam during the past few decades and are relatively common procedures nowadays. In Asia, many women patients, who have a round chin and square jaw, seek a softer and more feminine impression.[3] Techniques that are used in Asian facial bone contouring surgeries have been incorporated in the FFS and are the cornerstone of these procedures. Concomitant with advances in surgical techniques, improved anesthesia techniques and usage of devices such as oscillating saws greatly improved the quality of mandible contouring surgery. Both surgical time and blood loss significantly decreased for such cases. As a result, patients who would be required to spend their postoperative day in an ICU could be operated on an outpatient basis. All these factors furthered the popularity of facial bone contouring surgery.

[a] Dr Harrison H Lee Private Practice, 9301 Wilshire Boulevard, Suite 601, Beverly Hills, CA 90210, USA; [b] Facial Plastic Surgery- Private Practice, 620 Park Avenue, New York, NY 10065, USA
* Corresponding author.
E-mail address: beverlyhillssurgeon@yahoo.com

Otolaryngol Clin N Am 55 (2022) 859–870
https://doi.org/10.1016/j.otc.2022.04.006
0030-6665/22/© 2022 Elsevier Inc. All rights reserved.

JAW REDUCTION AS A PART OF FACIAL FEMINIZATION SURGERY

FFS began in 1982 when Dr Ed Falces who performed gender reassignment surgeries on transgender patients, approached Dr Douglas Ousterhout, a protégé of Dr Tessier, with a request from a transgender patient to make her face more feminine because people reacted to her as though she were a man. Up until then, Dr Ousterhout's practice predominantly involved craniofacial reconstruction of patients with birth defects, accidents, or other injuries. He conducted extensive research to identify which facial features would be identified as more feminine. He derived measurements defining those features from a series of cephalograms taken in the 1970s, and then worked with a set of several hundred skulls to determine if he could consistently differentiate women from men using those measurements only. He then began working out surgical techniques and materials in order to transform and feminize the male face.[4]

FFS, as a subspecialty of plastic surgery, was further revolutionized, and it became mainstream with refinement and improvement of techniques by the leaders and innovators of this field such as the senior author, Dr Harrison Lee. With his background as an oral maxillofacial surgeon coupled with ENT and Facial Plastic Surgery training, Dr Lee was uniquely placed to further the techniques of FFS. FFS performed on famous celebrity patients such as Caitlyn Jenner and Nikita Dragun by our senior author (HHL) also added to the popularity of this procedure.[5] In many of the cases, it is the first surgery undertaken by the patients who are transitioning from male to female. Our senior author (HHL) has extensive experience with FFS and has performed surgeries on more than 3000 patients during the past 20 years.

FFS necessitates a series of surgeries involving bone and soft tissue to alter the masculine features into a softer feminine appearance.[6] Jaw reduction is an integral and critical component of FFS. It is indicated for any transgender as well cis gender patients desiring a dramatic result by softening the square masculine jaw and prominent chin. In this article, we will focus on Jaw contouring procedures that are associated with FFS.

OVERALL DIFFERENCE IN MALE AND FEMALE JAW SKELETAL DIMENSIONS

The face plays a significant role in gender dysphoria seen in transgender patients. Gender dysphoria is currently diagnosed as per the World Professional Association for Transgender Health standard of care version 7.[7] It occurs in 1 in 30,000 male-assigned births and 1 in 100,000 female-assigned births.[8] There are prominent differences between the male and female facial anatomy, which can be altered surgically to alter the visual perception of the face.[9–11] In general, the biological male population has a wider, more square, and angular jaw. The masseter muscle tends to be more defined resulting in a strong jaw angle. The jaw line drops down and turns sharply giving a square appearance to the jaw. In women, it curves gently from earlobes to the chin.

JAW REDUCTION TECHNIQUE

It is highly recommended to get radiographic imaging as a part of the surgical planning. Besides Panorex X-ray, we also obtain a PA and lateral cephalogram routinely (**Fig. 1**). A 3D CT scan of the face can be obtained in lieu of or in addition to the plain films. Positioning of the mental nerve is noted in the imaging. The images are also carefully reviewed for any impacted teeth, any plates or screws from prior surgeries. An impacted tooth might need to be removed before the jaw reduction surgery.

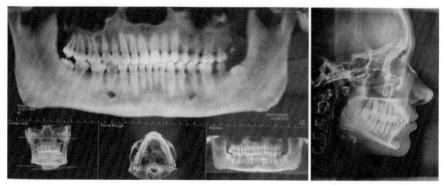

Fig. 1. Panorex X-rays and PA and Lateral Cephalogram of Jaw as a part of preoperative work up.

Our technique of jaw reduction involves sagittal resection of the mandible using a saw from the angle of the jaw to the mental nerve region (**Fig. 2**). This creates a smooth transition from the ramus to the chin and also retains the integrity of the inner portion of the mandible (**Fig. 3**). The anatomy of the gonial angle also plays a role in determining the extent of jaw reduction. If the gonial angle is flaring out, then the sagittal resection needs to go all the way to the angle of the mandible to address the gonial angle flaring. If the gonial angle is flaring inward, then it is possible to achieve optimal jaw contouring without aggressive resection. Specific attention is also given to the masseter muscle. It is not uncommon in biological male patients to have excessive or hypertrophied masseter muscle. Such patients benefit from concomitant resection of masseter muscles using electrocautery and bipolar to achieve an optimal result.

Another key point is addressing the soft tissue laxity that might arise from jaw reduction surgeries. With mandible resection, especially in patients with outward flaring gonial angle and hypertrophied masseter muscles, there is a significant risk of soft tissue laxity that might arise due to loss of bone structural support. Failure to address this can have an adverse effect on the overall outcome of the surgery. We, typically, combine these procedures with a neck lift and even, facelift depending on the extent of resection and the age and preoperative neck laxity of the patient. The extent of facelift and neck lift depends on the age and preop skin laxity of the patient and also depends on the extent of planned jaw reduction.

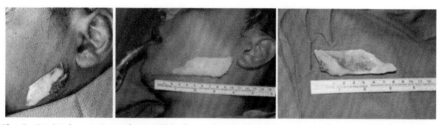

Fig. 2. Sagittal resection of mandible from the angle of the jaw to the mental nerve region for jaw reduction surgery.

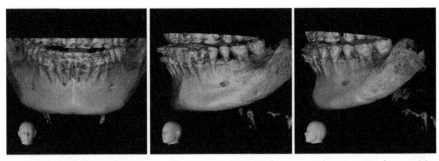

Fig. 3. Postoperative 3D CT scan after jaw reduction demonstrating a smooth transition from the mandible angle to the chin.

In our experience, we do not adhere to the usage of surgical templates. They tend to be inaccurate in dealing with the body of the mandible. They can be overly rigid and do not afford any artistic or surgical freedom. The template also does not guide with regards to soft tissue such as masseter muscle. In our purview, the gonial angle resection must be tailored to the individual patients and should not be the same for every patient. We will discuss a patient complication concerning template use in a subsequent portion of the article.

CHIN CONTOURING

Genioplasty and other chin contouring techniques have already been discussed in a separate article. However, our discussion of jaw reduction would be incomplete without a brief discussion on chin contouring. There are various ways to contour and soften the masculine chin. The chin can be shaved with a burr in selected cases. However, our preferred method for chin contouring is T-genioplasty. Male chin seems to be boxy, and a T-genioplasty technique with about 4 to 12 mm reduction of the central chin in the transverse direction can transform a boxy masculine chin into a softer feminine chin.

For T-genioplasty technique, we first mark the midline of the chin. If the facial midline is off from the chin midline, the facial midline needs to be transcribed to the chin midline. We then resect a predetermined amount of bone from the center of the chin as a part of the T-genioplasty, perform a horizontal osteotomy to mobilize the chin, remove the central portion, and then rigidly fix the chin with plates and screws (**Fig. 4**).

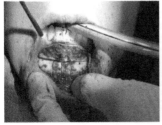
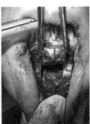
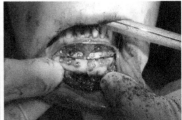

Fig. 4. Demonstration of T-genioplasty including resection of central chin and mobilization of chin components with plates and screws.

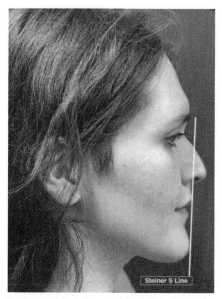 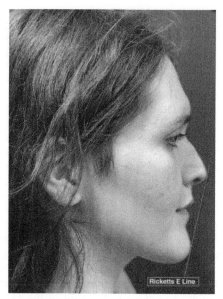

Fig. 5. Steiner S line and Ricketts E line to assess the A-P projection of the chin.

In terms of the A-P Projection of the chin, Steiner S Line and Ricketts E line can be used as a good reference (**Fig. 5**). Steiner S line connects the midpoint of the columella to the soft tissue pogonion. In an ideal projection, the upper and the lower lips should fall on this line and any deviation shows prominence or flatness of the chin. Ricketts E line is drawn from the nasal tip to the soft tissue pogonion. Ideally, the upper lip should be 5 mm behind and the lower lip should be 3 mm behind this line.

Another aspect of chin contouring involves alteration of the vertical proportion of the lower face. Ideally, the ratio of the upper lip length (Subnasale – upper lip stomion): the lower lip length (Lower lip stomion – menton) should be 1:2. As seen in this patient, the ratio is 1:2.6 (**Fig. 6**) with excess lower lip/chin length, which would need to be shortened to achieve ideal proportions.

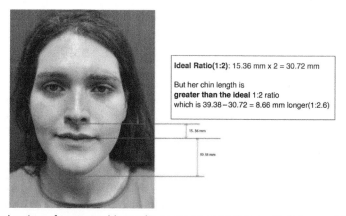

Ideal Ratio(1:2): 15.36 mm x 2 = 30.72 mm

But her chin length is
greater than the ideal 1:2 ratio
which is 39.38 – 30.72 = 8.66 mm longer(1:2.6)

15.36 mm

39.38 mm

Fig. 6. Ideal ration of upper and lower lip to assess vertical excess/deficiency of the chin.

GENERAL COMPLICATIONS

Overall, both jaw and chin contouring surgery are very safe with very low risks of complications when done correctly. However, there can be a myriad of potential complications that can arise from the surgery. Paresthesia or anesthesia along the distribution of inferior alveolar and mental nerve can be disconcerting to the patient. This is generally temporary but can be permanent in rare cases. Extreme care should be taken to avoid disruption of the mental nerve either due to traction injury or due to physical avulsion of the nerve during the surgery. We strongly recommend leaving a cuff of soft tissue around the mental nerve. Skeletonizing the mental nerve can make it prone to traction injury as well as increase the risk of avulsion injury. Damage to the marginal mandibular nerve can be of more significant concern and can occur when the periosteum is violated. We, therefore, very strongly recommend maintaining the surgery within the periosteal envelope. Violating the periosteal envelope posteriorly can also result in perforation of the retromandibular vein and more anteriorly—the facial vessels. Asymmetry of the jaw and the chin can be due to asymmetrical reduction or due to inability to address the preoperative asymmetry, based on clinical or radiological measurements, with differential reduction. Fracture of the mandible can occur as a complication during or after the surgery. Devitalization of the teeth can occur especially if you are too close to the root of the teeth. Another debilitating complication that can arise is ptosis of the chin a.k.a witch's chin. This is due to the failure to reapproximate mentalis muscle appropriately. Mentalis should always be reapproximated and realigned to avoid this complication.

Overresection of the mandible, chin, and masseter muscle can result in loss of soft tissue support. Integrity of soft tissue structures should always be assessed when performing jaw and chin reduction surgery. To address this, we perform submental and jaw line liposuction at the very minimum. However, we commonly add neck lift or facelift even in younger patients undergoing jaw reduction to address the loss of soft tissue support from the jaw reduction.

RESULTS

We have operated on more than 3000 patients during the past 20 years for FFS. Overall, our patients are extremely happy with their outcomes. We have included a few representative patients who underwent a combination of genioplasty and jaw reduction (**Fig. 7**). These pictures were taken between 3 and 24 months postoperative follow-up period. In our experience, jaw reduction surgery in combination with genioplasty is a very powerful tool to achieve optimal, precise, and reproducible results.

CASE STUDIES

We are also including 2 case studies of patients who were initially operated on by a different surgeon and required revision surgeries for varied reasons. We believe that there are major learning points in each case that would be very useful to the readers of this article.

Patient 1

The patient is a 39-year-old transgender female who underwent a T-genioplasty by another surgeon who used a preoperative surgical template to perform the surgery. Unfortunately, due to excessive narrowing of the chin with the template, the patient

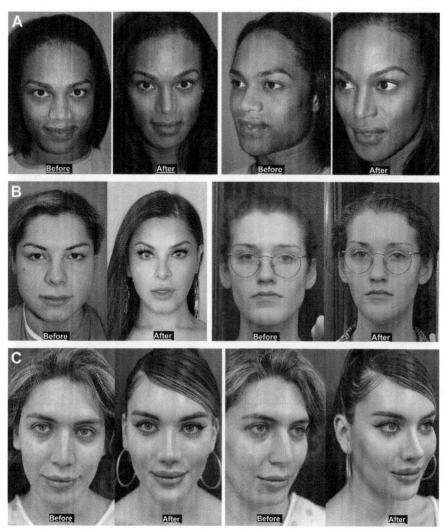

Fig. 7. (*A–C*): Postoperative outcomes of representative patients undergoing jaw reduction surgery and T-genioplasty as part of FFS. The average follow-up for these pictures are from 3 to 24 months.

developed an extremely narrow chin. She also had excess forward movement of the chin segments resulting in irregularities of the body of the mandible (**Fig. 8**). She was overall very unhappy with the results and sought revision surgery.

Her surgical correction included the removal of existing hardware, recreate the osteotomies to free up the chin segments, widen the chin complex with insertion of a cadaveric iliac crest graft, and lateralize the posterior aspects of the respective chin segments to align with the body of the mandible. We also resected step defect created by the genioplasty (**Fig. 9**). This resulted in significantly smooth transition from the chin to the jaw and significantly improved the appearance of the chin (**Fig. 10**). The biggest take away from this case is potential complications due to

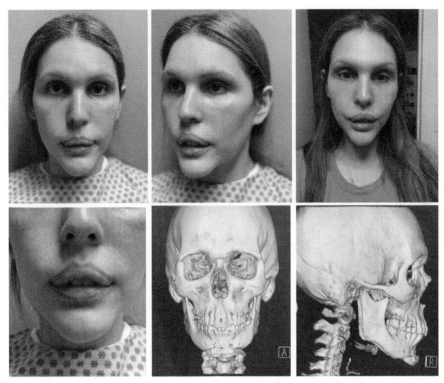

Fig. 8. Postoperative images and radiographic images of patient 1 after the initial surgery using surgical templates.

overreliance on templates. Although templates may serve as a guide for surgical planning, they cannot be used as a replacement for surgical expertise, assessment, and judgment.

Patient 2

The patient is a 31-year-old transgender female who underwent FFS by another surgeon. Unfortunately, her surgery involved overresection of mandible, chin, and masseter muscle. This resulted in loss of soft tissue support causing chin ptosis and neck laxity (**Fig. 11**). For her revision surgery, we did T-genioplasty to reapproximate her chin and suspended the chin pad to provide soft tissue support. We also added jaw angle implants to recreate her jaw angle and supported her cheeks with a cheek implant. Finally, face and neck lifts were done to address the laxity of her face and neck (**Fig. 12**). This resulted in significant smoothening of her chin and jaw line along with the improvement of neck laxity and chin ptosis.

There are multiple takeaways from this case. We should be extremely careful of being overzealous with bone and soft tissue resection. This can create a 2-fold problem. First, overresection can overcorrect the existing bone and soft tissue deformity and might require revision surgery. Second, careful attention should be given to neck and face laxity that might arise with jaw reduction. If this is not addressed appropriately, it results in significant neck laxity that would adversely affect the overall outcome.

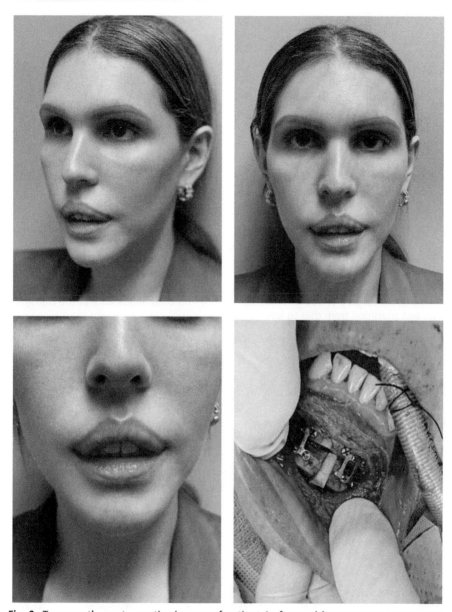

Fig. 9. Two months postoperative images of patient 1 after revision surgery at our center.

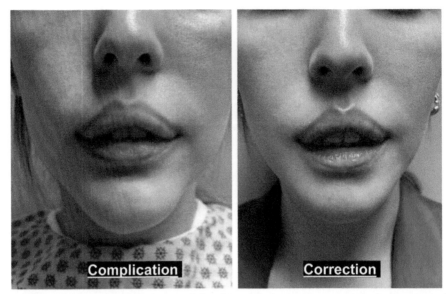

Fig. 10. Comparison of frontal view of the chin after the revision surgery when compared with the initial surgery. The patient has significantly improved appearance of the chin symmetry and transition from chin to jaw.

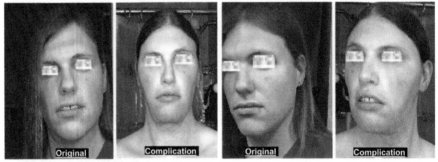

Fig. 11. Comparison of frontal and oblique view of patient 2 after initial surgery when compared with her preoperative pictures. She has loss of soft tissue support causing chin ptosis and neck laxity.

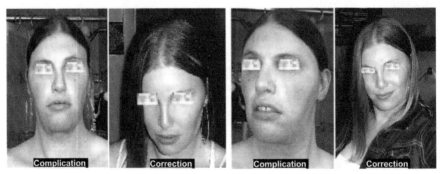

Fig. 12. Comparison of frontal view of patient 2 after the revision surgery when compared with initial surgery. She has significant smoothening of her chin and jaw line along with improvement of neck laxity and chin ptosis.

SUMMARY

Jaw reduction surgery, in combination with genioplasty, is a very powerful tool to alter the visual perception of the face. Our technique of jaw reduction involves sagittal resection of the mandible from the angle of the jaw to the mental nerve region. This creates a smooth transition from the ramus to the chin and also retains the integrity of the inner portion of the mandible. We have operated on more than 3000 patients during the past 20 years for FFS. Overall, our patients are extremely happy with their outcomes.

CLINICS CARE POINTS

- We strongly recommend a panorex X-ray, PA and Lateral cephalogram, and/or a 3D CT face for preoperative planning of jaw reduction surgery.
- Our technique of jaw reduction involves sagittal resection of mandible from the angle of the jaw to the mental nerve region.
- Our preferred method of chin contouring is T-genioplasty, which is generally done in combination with jaw reduction.
- We recommend to leave a cuff of soft tissue around the mental nerve during surgical dissection to minimize the risk of mental nerve injury.
- We very strongly recommend to maintain the surgery within the periosteal envelope to minimize the risk of injury to the retromandibular vein, facial vessels, and marginal mandibular nerve.
- Overresection of the mandible, chin, and soft tissue can result in the loss of soft tissue support and should be avoided.
- Consider a facelift/neck lift if there is concern of neck/face laxity secondary to jaw reduction. At minimum, liposuction of neck and chin should be performed in these cases.
- Overreliance on preoperative surgical templates can be deceptive and can lead to suboptimal outcomes.

DISCLOSURE

The authors have no commercial or financial conflicts of interest to declare. There was no funding for this study.

ACKNOWLEDGEMENTS

The authors would like to extend our most sincere appreciation to Sun Lee for her help in preparing the figures for this article and revising the article.

REFERENCES

1. Whitaker LA, Pertschuk M. Facial skeletal contouring for aesthetic purpose. Plast Reconstr Surg 1982;69(2):245–53.
2. Baek SM, kim SS, Bindiger A. The prominent mandibular angle: preoperative management, operative techniques, and results in 42 patients. Plast Reconstr Surg 1989;83(2):272–80.
3. Pu L. Aesthetic plastic surgery in Asians: Principles and techniques. Boca Raton: CRC; 2015.

4. Ousterhout DK. Feminization of the forehead: contour changing to improve female aesthetics. Plast Reconstr Surg 1987;79(05):701–13.
5. Singh M, Singh Chauhan A, Singh G, et al. Did Caitlyn Jenner's Facial Feminization Surgery Impact Public Interest in Gender Reassignment Surgery and Facial Feminization Surgery? Facial Plast Surg Aesthet Med 2020;22(2):117–9.
6. Capitán L, Simon D, Kaye K, et al. Facial feminization surgery: the forehead. Surgical techniques and analysis of results. Plast Reconstr Surg 2014;134(04):609–19.
7. Coleman E, Bockting W, Botzer M, et al. Standards of care for the health of transsexual, transgender, and gender-nonconforming people, Version 7. Int J Transgenderism 2011;134:165–232.
8. Gender identity disorders. In: Marcov itch H, editor. Black's Medical Dictionary 43rd edLondon. A&C Black; 2018. p. 290.
9. Becking AG, Tuinzing DB, Hage JJ, et al. Facial corrections in male to female transsexuals: a preliminary report on 16 patients. J Oral Maxillofac Surg 1996;54(04):413–8.
10. Hage JJ, Becking AG, de Graaf FH, et al. Gender-confirming facial surgery: considerations on the masculinity and femininity of faces. Plast Reconstr Surg 1997;99(07):1799–807.
11. Spiegel JH. Facial determinants of female gender and feminizing forehead cranioplasty. Laryngoscope 2011;121(2):250–61.

Chondrolaryngoplasty

Christopher G. Tang, MD[a], Peter M. Debbaneh, MD[b],
Andrew J. Kleinberger, MD[c],*

KEYWORDS

- Chondrolaryngoplasty • Tracheal shave • Feminizing laryngoplasty • Transgender
- Facial feminization

KEY POINTS

- Chondrolaryngoplasty is a surgical procedure often performed as part of facial feminization surgery for transgender patients with a diagnosis of gender dysphoria.
- When performed with direct visualization of the vocal cords by using a flexible fiberoptic scope placed through a laryngeal mask airway (LMA), chondrolaryngoplasty can be completed efficiently with maximal thyroid cartilage resection and minimal risk of laryngeal injury.
- Chondrolaryngoplasty has been demonstrated to lead to high rates of postoperative satisfaction and improvements in overall quality of life.
- Alternatives to the traditional transcervical approach such as submental and transoral techniques may provide for improved aesthetic outcomes and should be further investigated.

HISTORY AND BACKGROUND

Chondrolaryngoplasty, or laryngeal chondroplasty as first described in the literature by Wolfort and Parry in 1975,[1] has gained increasing recognition as a procedure aimed to address a marked anatomic source of gender dysphoria in transgender patients as well as for general aesthetic purposes. The initial surgical technique was described as an open transcervical approach through an incision directly overlying the thyroid notch. A perichondrial incision was then made along the superior border of the outer lamina to access the thyroid cartilage.

Wolfort later published a modified description of his technique in 1990 that involves the addition of a burr for contour refinement after cartilage resection.[2] He reported that of the 31 patients undergoing this procedure since 1972, 21 exhibited postoperative

[a] Department of Head and Neck Surgery, Kaiser Permanente Medical Center at San Francisco, 450 6th Avenue 2nd Floor, San Francisco, CA 94118, USA; [b] Department of Head and Neck Surgery, Kaiser Permanente Medical Center at Oakland, 3600 Broadway, 4th Floor, Oakland, CA 94611, USA; [c] Department of Head and Neck Surgery, Kaiser Permanente Medical Center at Walnut Creek, 1425 South Main Street, 3rd Floor, Walnut Creek, CA 94596, USA
* Corresponding author.
E-mail address: andrew.j.kleinberger@kp.org

Otolaryngol Clin N Am 55 (2022) 871–884
https://doi.org/10.1016/j.otc.2022.04.009
0030-6665/22/© 2022 Elsevier Inc. All rights reserved.

voice disturbances that in one case lasted up to 6 months. In an effort to reduce the risk of vocal cord injury, a subsequent technique was developed during which direct laryngoscopy was used to evaluate the precise location of the vocal cords before thyroid cartilage resection.[3] Spiegel and colleagues expanded on this concept in 2008 by incorporating the use of a laryngeal mask airway (LMA) combined with flexible fiberoptic laryngoscopy.[4] This now widely used bronchoscopic-assisted chondrolaryngoplasty technique involves intraoperative needle localization of the anterior commissure to aid in determining the precise extent of thyroid cartilage resection.

LARYNGEAL ANATOMY

The larynx is a cartilaginous organ of the respiratory tract located in the anterior neck that functions to provide phonation and protect the lower airways. Development begins at week 4 of intrauterine life as the laryngotracheal groove, which divides into an anterior respiratory system and posterior esophagus by the esophagotracheal septum at around week 5. There is initially little variation between male and female larynges until puberty, during which time the male larynx grows considerably larger, particularly in the anteroposterior dimension. On average, the larynx is 36 mm in men and 26 mm in women. Functionally, this embryologic and anatomic difference translates into the typically observed deeper male voice.

The laryngeal skeleton is comprised of the hyoid bone and 3 paired cartilages including the arytenoid, corniculate, and cuneiform cartilages as well as 3 unpaired cartilages including the thyroid cartilage, cricoid cartilage, and epiglottis. The thyroid cartilage is the largest element of the larynx and has a shield-like shape, with both thyroid lamina meeting at the midline to form a superior protrusion known as the laryngeal prominence or thyroid notch. This external landmark, commonly referred to as the Adam's apple, is the primary target of the chondrolaryngoplasty procedure (**Fig. 1**).

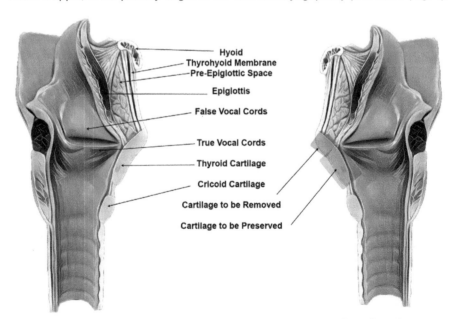

Hyoid
Thyrohyoid Membrane
Pre-Epiglottic Space

Epiglottis

False Vocal Cords

True Vocal Cords

Thyroid Cartilage

Cricoid Cartilage

Cartilage to be Removed

Cartilage to be Preserved

Fig. 1. Diagram of cross-sectional laryngeal anatomy demonstrating thyroid cartilage resection. (*From* Tang CG. Evaluating patient benefit from laryngochondroplasty. Laryngoscope. 130:S1-S14, 2020; with permission.)

The larynx is bordered by the sternocleidomastoid muscles laterally and lies deep into the platysma and strap muscles. During a transcervical approach, these muscles are typically separated at the midline and retracted laterally to access the thyroid cartilage.

The internal space of the larynx, which is lined by mucosa, can be divided into 3 anatomic subunits: the supraglottis (including the epiglottis and arytenoids), glottis (both true and false vocal cords as well as the laryngeal ventricles in between them), and subglottis (space just below the glottis). The internal portion of the larynx is wider superiorly, with the glottis being the most narrow part in adults. Several important structures attach to the inner surface of the thyroid cartilage including the epiglottis superiorly, followed by the ventricular or false vocal folds, extending from the bodies of the arytenoid cartilages posteriorly to the thyroid cartilage anteriorly. The true vocal folds or cords attach to the thyroid cartilage inferior to the ventricular folds and consist of a musculomembranous portion within the anterior three-fifths of the cord and a cartilaginous portion within the posterior two-fifths of the cord, formed by the vocal process of the arytenoid cartilage.[5] Just inferior to the attachment of the thyroepiglottic ligament, the bilateral true vocal cords insert into the internal lamina of the thyroid cartilage at the anterior commissure. Once identified by needle localization, the portion of thyroid cartilage superior to this point can be safely removed without causing laryngeal injury (**Fig. 2**).

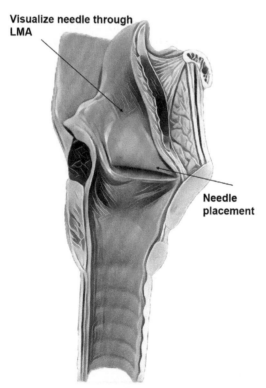

Fig. 2. Diagram of cross-sectional laryngeal anatomy demonstrating vocal cord localization. (*From* Tang CG. Evaluating patient benefit from laryngochondroplasty. Laryngoscope. 130:S1-S14, 2020; with permission.)

The laryngeal blood supply is provided by the superior and inferior laryngeal arteries, branches of the superior thyroid artery and inferior thyroid artery, respectively. The superior laryngeal artery enters the larynx through the thyrohyoid membrane along with the internal branch of the superior laryngeal nerve. The inferior laryngeal artery ascends the trachea and enters the larynx with the recurrent laryngeal nerve. The larynx receives both motor and sensory innervation from the vagus nerve (cranial nerve X) via the superior and recurrent laryngeal nerves. The superior laryngeal nerve travels between the internal and external carotid vessels and separates just below the hyoid into the internal branch, which enters the larynx through the thyrohyoid membrane to supply sensation to the mucosa of the larynx, and the external branch, which innervates the cricothyroid muscle. The recurrent laryngeal nerve innervates all intrinsic muscles of the larynx, except the cricothyroid muscle, with varying side-dependent courses.

EVALUATION

The preoperative evaluation is a critical aspect of ensuring successful surgical outcomes after chondrolaryngoplasty. The main goal is to maximize overall postoperative satisfaction through appropriate patient selection and a thorough discussion of potential risks and expectations.

Patient Selection and Expectations of Surgery

Appropriate patient selection and a thorough review of expectations are essential elements of the preoperative consultation. Ideally, patients should initially be evaluated by a multidisciplinary health care team including medical and mental health providers before surgery referral. Candidacy for chondrolaryngoplasty should be determined based on several factors including overall medical and psychological well-being, reasonability of expectations, and physical examination findings. As can be seen from **Fig. 3**, there is a wide range of neck anatomy that may be encountered during preoperative evaluation, and the degree of improvement after chondrolaryngoplasty can vary considerably. For instance, a patient with a slender neck and relatively large thyroid cartilage will likely have a more impactful outcome when compared with a patient with smaller thyroid cartilage and overlying submental liposis. It is important to note that the degree of dysphoria does not necessarily correlate proportionately with the degree of Adam's apple visibility. There are patients with significant dysphoria and rather subtle appearing laryngeal landmarks, as well as those with highly prominent thyroid cartilage not interested in pursuing surgery. As a general rule, if the postoperative neck scar is likely to be more visible than the cartilage itself and/or the cartilage does not break the plane of the overall neck contour and protrude on profile, deferring surgery may be prudent. Additionally, due to anatomic constraints, a completely smooth cervical contour may not be possible and a residual, albeit smaller, cartilaginous prominence may persist in some cases postoperatively (**Fig. 4**). Occasionally the most visible laryngeal landmark may actually be the cricoid cartilage and pointing this out when managing expectations is important. Preoperative patient selection and detailed counseling based on these factors are critical to optimizing surgical outcomes.

Preoperative Evaluation

The preoperative evaluation should include 3 main elements: (1) physical examination (including voice assessment), (2) photographic documentation of the patient's neck, and (3) thorough discussion of the risks, benefits, and limitations of the procedure.

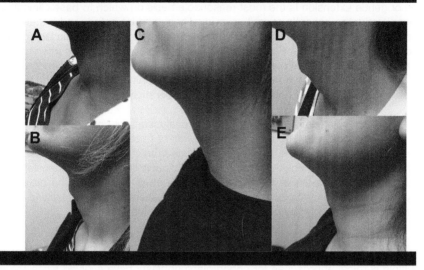

Fig. 3. *A-E:* Variety of neck anatomy seen during preoperative evaluation for chondrolaryngoplasty. (*From* Tang CG. Evaluating patient benefit from laryngochondroplasty. Laryngoscope. 130:S1-S14, 2020; with permission.)

A focused physical examination of the neck should be performed noting the degree of thyroid cartilage prominence, overlying skin quality and overall neck habitus, and presence of a cervicomental crease or preexisting neck scars. The neck should be examined from multiple views in both a neutral position as well as an extension during which the cartilage will typically become accentuated. Since in far extension, even a

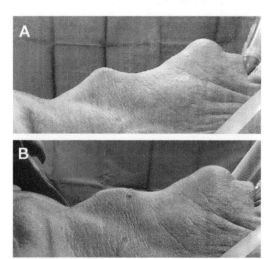

Fig. 4. Preoperative (*A*) and postoperative (*B*) photographs showing profile view of thyroid cartilage reduction and residual prominence after chondrolaryngoplasty. (*From* Tang CG. Evaluating patient benefit from laryngochondroplasty. Laryngoscope. 130:S1-S14, 2020; with permission.)

rather subtle appearing thyroid cartilage may seem significant, the neutral neck position or gentle extension is the most reasonable basis on which to base clinical decisions. Lastly, the patient's overall voice quality should be noted, and if there is any dysphonia or history of vocal disturbance, an in-office flexible fiberoptic laryngoscopy should be performed. Some surgeons, as with thyroid or parathyroid surgery, may opt to perform a preoperative diagnostic laryngoscopy routinely for all patients undergoing chondrolaryngoplasty to detect any preexisting laryngeal pathology or functional conditions that may be present in case a postoperative voice complication were to arise.

Another key element of the preoperative evaluation for chondrolaryngoplasty is photographic documentation. A standard series of photographs should be taken of the neck including up to the cervicomental angle from multiple perspectives. The patient's neck should be positioned in a neutral position as well as in extension during which the thyroid cartilage will typically become more prominent. The presence of any significant neck pathology such as preexisting scars, cutaneous lesions, rhytids, or asymmetry of the laryngeal landmarks should also be noted.

SURGICAL TECHNIQUE

Multiple surgical approaches for chondrolaryngoplasty have evolved since the procedure's inception in the 1970s. We will first discuss in detail the bronchoscopic-assisted localization technique currently used by the authors and originally described by Spiegel and colleagues in 2008.[4]

Anesthesia and Operating Room Setup

A functioning flexible fiberoptic bronchoscope and display monitor should be positioned on the left-hand side of the OR table to allow for optimal anesthesia access and surgeon viewing. The patient is then brought into the room and laid in a standard supine position. Following the routine timeout protocol and induction of general anesthesia, a Teleflex Classic (Teleflex, Westmeath, Ireland) or similar LMA size 4 or 5 (**Fig. 5**) is carefully placed and secured with the patient's neck slightly extended. The planned incision within or above the cervicomental junction can be marked at this point or alternatively with the patient sitting up in the preoperative area (**Fig. 6**).

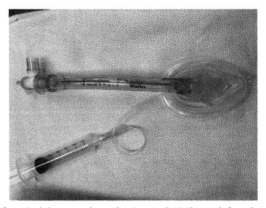

Fig. 5. Example of typical laryngeal mask airway (LMA) used for chondrolaryngoplasty. (*From* Tang CG. Evaluating patient benefit from laryngochondroplasty. Laryngoscope. 130:S1-S14, 2020; with permission.)

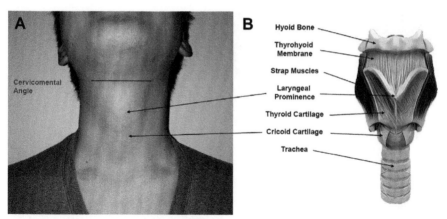

Fig. 6. External view of the laryngeal prominence (*A*) corresponding to (*B*) anatomic depiction of laryngeal structures. (*From* Tang CG. Evaluating patient benefit from laryngochondroplasty. Laryngoscope. 130:S1-S14, 2020; with permission.)

As the incision placement moves superiorly toward the submental region, additional downward retraction and possibly incision length will be needed for visualization. Local anesthesia is then infiltrated along the planned incision site and overlying the thyroid cartilage. The patient is then prepped and draped in a sterile fashion, exposing the neck while leaving the anesthesia provider access to the LMA to perform intraoperative laryngoscopy.

Operative Technique

An approximately 2 cm transverse incision is made with a 15 blade through the skin, dermis, and subcutaneous tissue. Blunt dissection is performed overlying the thyroid cartilage to the level of the platysma or investing layer of deep cervical fascia, which is then divided horizontally. Strap muscles are identified and divided at the midline raphe. The strap muscles are then retracted laterally to expose the thyroid cartilage in "key-hole" fashion (**Fig. 7**). Bovie electrocautery can be used to carefully make an incision through the outer thyroid lamina perichondrium along the superior margin which is then gently elevated from the cartilage inferiorly with a Freer elevator.

At this point, the anesthesia provider is asked to place the bronchoscope through the LMA to visualize the vocal cords. A 22-gauge needle is then inserted through the thyroid lamina in the midline approximately at the junction between the upper third and lower two-thirds of the thyroid cartilage to identify the location of the anterior commissure (**Fig. 8**). This intraoperative localization technique allows for the maximal amount of thyroid cartilage to be resected while preventing damage to the vocal cords or the thyroepiglottic ligament. Once the proper location is confirmed, this level is marked externally along the thyroid cartilage with Bovie electrocautery and the needle and bronchoscope are then withdrawn (**Fig. 9**). Using a rongeur, the cartilage superior to this point is then carefully removed, typically starting with a paramedian segment and avoiding any mucosal tears. The thyroid cartilage can also be excised with an en bloc technique (**Figs. 10** and **11**). As described by Wolfort, Conrad and Spiegel, great care must be taken to only remove the cartilage superior to the initial marking.[1–4] The remaining cartilage should be assessed for symmetry and any palpable irregularities that can be smoothed with a rongeur or electrocautery on cutting mode. The field is then irrigated well and hemostasis is obtained. Bronchoscopy should be repeated to confirm the integrity of the anterior commissure.

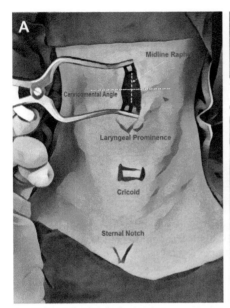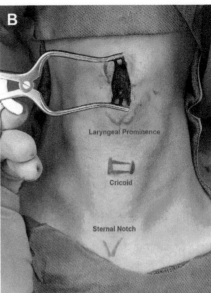

Fig. 7. Anatomic depiction of intraoperative exposure of the thyroid cartilage through a cervicomental incision (*A*) and intraoperative photograph (*B*). (*From* Tang CG. Evaluating patient benefit from laryngochondroplasty. Laryngoscope. 130:S1-S14, 2020; with permission.)

A meticulous layered closure is then performed starting with the reapproximation of the strap muscles vertically in the midline. Care should be taken to avoid injury to the anterior jugular veins as well as to ensure there is no tethering of the muscles to the underlying cartilage. The platysma and deep subcutaneous tissues should then be closed followed by a running subcuticular stitch or skin glue. No surgical drains are typically necessary (see **Fig. 4**; **Fig. 12**).

Technique Variations

Before using endoscopic techniques for precise intraoperative vocal cord localization, chondrolaryngoplasty had been performed by approximating the amount of thyroid cartilage that can be safely removed based on the height of the thyroid cartilage. While possibly leading to favorable results in some cases, this approach has the potential for

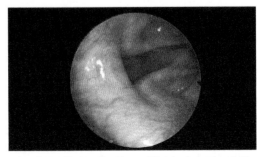

Fig. 8. Endoscopic-assisted needle localization of the laryngeal anterior commissure. (*From* Tang CG. Evaluating patient benefit from laryngochondroplasty. Laryngoscope. 130:S1-S14, 2020; with permission.)

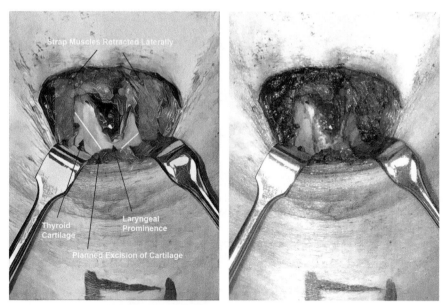

Fig. 9. Anatomic depiction of intraoperative demarcation of planned thyroid cartilage resection (A) and intraoperative photograph (B) (*From* Tang CG. Evaluating patient benefit from laryngochondroplasty. Laryngoscope. 130:S1-S14, 2020; with permission.)

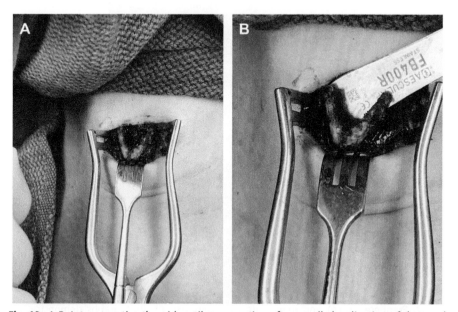

Fig. 10. A-B: Intraoperative thyroid cartilage resection after needle localization of the vocal cords. (*From* Tang CG. Evaluating patient benefit from laryngochondroplasty. Laryngoscope. 130:S1-S14, 2020; with permission.)

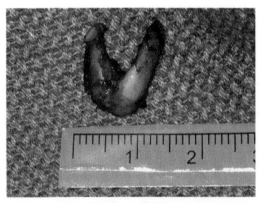

Fig. 11. Example of superior portion of thyroid cartilage excised after en bloc resection technique. (*From* Tang CG. Evaluating patient benefit from laryngochondroplasty. Laryngoscope. 130:S1-S14, 2020; with permission.)

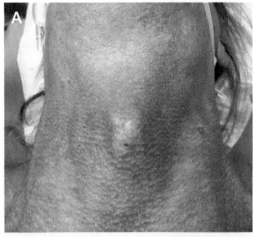

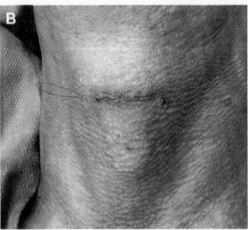

Fig. 12. Preoperative (*A*) and immediate postoperative (*B*) photographs demonstrating change in frontal view of neck after thyroid cartilage reduction. (*From* Tang CG. Evaluating patient benefit from laryngochondroplasty. Laryngoscope. 130:S1-S14, 2020; with permission.)

both cartilage under resection due to conservative underestimation or over resection with an increased risk of laryngeal injury. Aesthetic and voice outcomes reliability improved with the introduction of intraoperative localization techniques to facilitate a more accurate thyroid cartilage excision.

Cartilage resection can be performed with several instruments based on surgeon preference and tissue quality including rongeur, scalpel, electrocautery, or powered drill. Softer cartilage may be readily excised sharply or by electrocautery, while partially ossified cartilage, as often seen in older patients, may necessitate the use of a rongeur or drill. Additional protection of the internal perichondrium with either a fine malleable or forceps has been described while using an 11 blade.[6] Postexcision smoothing and contouring have been described with a burr,[2] Bovie electrocautery on cutting, or with an 11 blade to make shearing cuts on the outer lamina.[7]

More recent minimally invasive chondrolaryngoplasty techniques include the submental and transoral or "scarless" approach. Inspired by transoral thyroid and parathyroid surgery, studies have described an incision made through the midline oral vestibule, between the mental nerves, with subperiosteal and subplatysmal dissection to the hyoid and thyroid cartilages.[8] In the original technique reported by Kafif and colleagues, the level of the anterior commissure was determined by transillumination using a bronchoscope through the laryngeal lumen. None of the 4 patients included in this study had any reported postoperative voice complications.[9]

COMPLICATIONS

Postoperative complications after chondrolaryngoplasty are rare and can include scarring (**Fig. 13**), bleeding and hematoma, or a disturbance in laryngeal function. History of atypical scarring should be discussed in detail, particularly for patients with hypertrophic scars or keloids. While skin incisions were initially placed directly overlying the laryngeal prominence, modern approaches try to camouflage the incision within or above the cervicomental angle. In addition to incision placement, closure technique is also important to reduce the risk of postoperative scarring and soft tissue tethering. It is critical to ensure the strap muscles are adequately reapproximated in the midline over the residual thyroid cartilage to prevent the development of adhesions to the

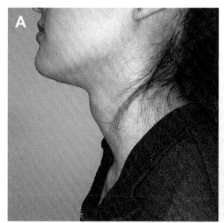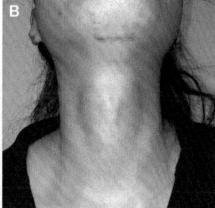

Fig. 13. Example of hypertrophic scarring of a submental incision after chondrolaryngoplasty. (*From* Tang CG. Evaluating patient benefit from laryngochondroplasty. Laryngoscope. 130:S1-S14, 2020; with permission.)

overlying skin. This may manifest as visible dimpling or bunching of the skin and subcutaneous tissues of the anterior neck particularly with dynamic laryngeal elevation during swallowing. Management of this complication should initially consist of conservative measures such as manual massage and typically tends to resolve over time.

Bleeding or hematoma formation is particularly concerning because of the proximity to the airway and potential for airway edema. While early reports of chondrolaryngoplasty describe the placement of surgical drains, routine use is no longer considered necessary. Following trends in thyroid and parathyroid surgery, the procedure can typically be performed in the outpatient setting. Postoperative monitoring may be indicated for longer facial feminization procedures.

Postoperative dysphagia has been observed in a small percentage of patients. Lee and colleagues found that 5 out of 88 (5.7%) patients surveyed after chondrolaryngoplasty reported mild swallowing difficulties, yet only 2 of these 5 attributed their symptoms to the actual surgery.[10] Identifying clear causation may also be confounded by throat symptoms commonly associated with LMA placement and/or intubation as well as that reported by the general population.

Voice outcomes have dramatically improved since the introduction of needle localization techniques. For example, Wolfort and colleagues reported a 65% rate of postoperative hoarseness or voice weakness, which generally resolved in less than 20 days. However, in one patient, voice changes persisted for 6 months.[2] In comparison, no significant voice complications were reported in 31 patients undergoing chondrolaryngoplasty with the bronchoscopic-assisted technique described by Spiegel and colleagues[4] Laryngeal injury may not only lead to deeper voice quality and worsening of gender dysphoria, but can also be difficult to treat and is best avoided.

DISCUSSION

Chondrolaryngoplasty was described almost 50 years ago as a surgical procedure aimed at reducing the prominence of the thyroid cartilage or Adam's apple. Technology-driven modifications to this initially presented technique have helped to improve overall efficacy and safety. Central to this evolution was the incorporation of the flexible fiberoptic bronchoscope to provide intraoperative visualization of the vocal cords. This now commonly used approach affords the operating surgeon the confidence to maximally remove the excess or nonsupportive superior portion of the thyroid cartilage with the preservation of laryngeal integrity and function.

While chondrolaryngoplasty can be performed for any individual seeking an aesthetic reduction in thyroid cartilage prominence, this procedure is currently most commonly used for transgender patients with a diagnosis of gender dysphoria. Chondrolaryngoplasty can be performed by itself or in conjunction with other facial feminization procedures. Proper patient selection and preoperative counseling, ideally carried out in collaboration with a multidisciplinary health care team experienced with gender-affirming surgeries, is critical to optimizing patients' outcomes. A long-term study by van de Grift and colleagues looked at postoperative satisfaction 4 to 6 years after first clinical contact in 236 transgender patients undergoing gender-affirming surgeries and showed that overall satisfaction was 94% to 100%, depending on the type of surgery performed. The 8 patients (6%) in the study who were dissatisfied with their surgery in long-term follow-up were associated with either self-reported surgical complications or preoperative psychological symptoms.[11] Several other studies have demonstrated high rates of postoperative satisfaction and improvements in overall quality of life specifically following chondrolaryngoplasty.[7,12,13]

Chondrolaryngoplasty can typically be performed on an outpatient basis, with inpatient monitoring reserved for patients with otherwise difficult airways, medical comorbidities, or those undergoing longer combined surgical procedures. The incidence of both short and long-term complications after surgery is low with the most commonly observed complaints pertaining to scar appearance and persistent thyroid cartilage prominence. Long-term voice and swallowing issues are rarely encountered, particularly when the vocal cords are visualized intraoperatively. Transoral approaches have been described that potentially eliminate the risks associated with postoperative scarring. Future studies are needed to more rigorously evaluate the safety profile and efficacy of these procedures as compared with the more traditional transcervical technique.

SUMMARY

Chondrolaryngoplasty is a now widely performed procedure that provides a reduction in thyroid cartilage prominence. The most common indication is for patients with a diagnosis of gender dysphoria, often performed as part of more comprehensive facial feminization surgery. Intraoperative localization of the vocal cords is paramount in determining the extent of thyroid cartilage resection and minimizing the risk of laryngeal injury. Overall, chondrolaryngoplasty has a favorable safety profile and leads to high rates of postoperative satisfaction and improvement in quality of life.

CLINICS CARE POINTS

- Chondrolaryngoplasty is a safe and effective procedure with high satisfaction rates in patients with gender dysphoria.

- Appropriate patient selection and preoperative counseling are important aspects of optimizing surgical outcomes.

- Intraoperative visualization of the vocal cords is critical to ensure maximal thyroid cartilage reduction with the preservation of laryngeal function.

- Postoperative complications after chondrolaryngoplasty are rare including long-term risks of postoperative dysphagia and dysphonia.

- Further studies are needed to compare the safety profile and outcomes of more recently described transoral techniques with traditional transcervical approaches.

DISCLOSURE

Support for portions of this work was provided by the Permanente Medical Group Delivery Science and Applied Research Program. The authors have no other funding, financial relationships, or conflicts of interest to disclose.

REFERENCES

1. Wolfort FG, Parry RG. Laryngeal chondroplasty for appearance. Plast Reconstr Surg 1975;56(4):371–4.
2. Wolfort FG, Dejerine ES, Ramos DJ, et al. Chondrolaryngoplasty for appearance. Plast Reconstr Surg 1990;86(3):464–9 [discussion: 470].
3. Conrad K, Yoskovitch A. Endoscopically facilitated reduction laryngochondroplasty. Arch Facial Plast Surg 2003;5(4):345–8.

4. Spiegel JH, Rodriguez G. Chondrolaryngoplasty under general anesthesia using a flexible fiberoptic laryngoscope and laryngeal mask airway. Arch Otolaryngol Head Neck Surg 2008;134(7):704–8.

5. Janfaza P, Montgomery WW, Randolph GW. Anterior regions of the neck. In: Janfaza P, Nadol JB Jr, Galla R, et al, editors. Surgical anatomy of the head and neck. 2nd edition. Cambridge (MA): Harvard University Press; 2011. p. 636–53.

6. Giraldo F, de Grado J, Montes J. Aesthetic reductive thyroid chondroplasty. Int J Oral Maxillofac Surg 1997;26(1):20–2.

7. Therattil PJ, Hazim NY, Cohen WA, et al. Esthetic reduction of the thyroid cartilage: a systematic review of chondrolaryngoplasty. JPRAS Open 2019;22:27–32.

8. Chung J, Purnell P, Anderson S, et al. Transoral chondrolaryngoplasty: scarless reduction of the Adam's apple. OTO Open 2020;4(3):1–3.

9. Khafif A, Shoffel-Havakuk H, Yaish I, et al. Scarless neck feminization: transoral transvestibular approach chondrolaryngoplasty. Facial Plast Surg Aesthet Med 2020;22(3):172–80.

10. Lee A, Wisco JJ, Shehan JN, et al. Dysphagia after gender affirming chondrolaryngoplasty (Tracheal Shave): A Survey Study. Facial Plast Surg Aesthet Med 2021. https://doi.org/10.1089/fpsam.2021.0214.

11. van de Grift TC, Elaut E, Cerwenka SC, et al. Surgical satisfaction, quality of life, and their association after gender-affirming surgery: a follow-up study. J Sex Marital Ther 2018;44(2):138–48.

12. Cohen MB, Insalaco LF, Tonn CR, et al. Patient Satisfaction after Aesthetic Chondrolaryngoplasty. Plast Reconstr Surg Glob Open 2018;6(10):e1877.

13. Tang CG. Evaluating patient benefit from laryngochondroplasty. Laryngoscope 2020;130:S1–14.

Three-Dimensional Planning in Hairline Surgery of Transgender Patients

Anna V. Sluzky, MD[a],*, Anastasiya V. Lyubchenko, MD[b],
Aina M. Magomedova, MD[c]

KEYWORDS

- Transgender surgery • Hairline surgery • Feminization surgery • Facial feminization
- 3D modeling

KEY POINTS

- Hairline growth pattern has an important role in gender identefication.
- Usage of three-dimensional modeling in preoperative stage significantly helps for surgeon in planning of future result and for discussion about patient expectations.
- There's no need to buy expensive equipment to introduce three-dimensional planning in your clinical practise: most tools can be used by your cell phone.

INTRODUCTION

The representation of a woman face includes many different points, one of which is the hair pattern, which is an important characteristic of gender identification. Here we describe our use of three-dimensional (3D) modeling methods in perioperative planning.

AIM

The aim of this study is to investigate and evaluate 3D modeling prospects in the hairline surgery of transgender patients.

BACKGROUND

One of the less obvious but important parts of facial structures that allows us to differentiate between women and men is the hairline pattern. An M-shaped hairline and a

---

[a] Kiriat-Haim, Israel, Haifa, Khoma U Migdal Street 44; [b] Department of Oncology, Radiotherapy and Plastic Surgery, I.M. Sechenov First Moscow State Medical University, 119991 Moscow, Trubetskaya Street, House 8, Building 2, Russia; [c] FACEMAKER, Chongarskiy Bulvar 5, 117452 Moscow, Russia
* Corresponding author.
E-mail address: sluzky@yandex.ru

Otolaryngol Clin N Am 55 (2022) 885–890
https://doi.org/10.1016/j.otc.2022.05.003
0030-6665/22/© 2022 Elsevier Inc. All rights reserved.

oto.theclinics.com

sloping forehead are typically associated with a man face and require surgical treatment to get a more feminine and natural look.

METHODS

We include male-to-female transgender patients who underwent hairline surgery as part of facial feminization surgery with and without perioperative 3D planning. Patient satisfaction was also assessed using a satisfaction questionnaire that they complete after a 6-month postoperative period.

CONCLUSION

Hairline surgery as part of facial feminization surgery is very important.

The use of 3D modeling at the level of preoperative preparation makes it possible to achieve greater compliance between the surgeon and the patient, to obtain a more aesthetically pleasing result.

BACKGROUND

It is generally accepted that it takes only a few seconds to distinguish between men and women faces. The visual identification of facial gender is one of the social and behavioral abilities of our brain set into action by activating a neural system that encompasses the main areas of the visual cortex, as well as the expanded limbic and prefrontal areas.[1] The part of the brain that is responsible for face recognition grows throughout life. Though differences in the speed and quality of men and women face differentiation are an object of many studies, a common tendency still exits: face recognition is a fast process, which occurs by reading certain facial proportions corresponding to a particular gender.

Gender identity and the level of gender dysphoria are greatly influenced by 3 main aspects: reflection in the mirror, surrounding society, and photo rating apps. To recognize a person's gender, one needs 0.03 seconds. Transgender patients experience some difficulty in social interactions as identification may exceed this time. If the duration of eye contact exceeds the socially acceptable average, the person acting as the object of visual identification experiences increased levels of anxiety. In the case of transgender patients, this may amplify gender dysphoria.

The vast majority of transgender patients are in the process of hormone replacement therapy, so we recommend conducting a genetic analysis (androgen receptor gene polymorphism and selected estrogen receptor) to determine androgen receptors susceptibility. By determining the level of androgen receptor susceptibility, it is possible to predict whether there will be a positive/effective result from hormone therapy.

All facial features provide some gender information. Their recognition and classification are related to our stereotypical patterns. A very important factor that determines the masculinity/femininity of the face is the upper third of the face, especially the frontal-naso-orbital complex and the hairline. sourse 2 The testosterone hormone induces male facial features such as increased supraorbital ridges, heavier low-set eyebrows, a protruding nasal angle, deeper orbits, an M-shaped hairline, a wide nose, flat cheeks, a square chin and jaw, as well as a flattened surface compared with the average female forehead. Hair, the hairline pattern, facial hair, skin texture, and the distribution and volume of facial fat give us a complete picture of a person's gender perception.[2]

The importance of the hairline pattern is not obvious, but according to some authors, the upper third of the face, especially the hairline pattern, is the second important feature of gender.[1-3] Thus, focusing on the upper third of the face, the thickness and degree of protrusion of the brow ridges, the observer is able to determine the gender of a person.[3] There are some gender parameters of the hairline and the hair pattern: *height of the hairline*, that is, the distance between the glabella and the trichion (intersection of the hairline and the midline of the forehead); *hair density*–the number of follicular units per square centimeter on the scalp. Typically, the male hairline is 7 to 8 cm above the glabella, and 5 to 7 cm in women. This distance is different for men and women; we should strive for these parameters.[4–17] sourse 18

There are various techniques for correcting the hairline of transgender women.[8,10,13–16] The basic principle of MtF Surgery is to lower the hairline and round the shape, moving away as far as possible from the "M–shape" characteristic of men. Hairline design in women is quite complex; there are endless variations. The only recurring theme is that the hairline should not be very even. The hairline and the ratio of the forehead to the face are important elements for making an attractive face. When the hairline is disrupted, the overall balance of the face changes (**Fig. 1**).

There are several risk factors for unacceptable scar formation after surgery. These include excessive tension, incorrect matching of the wound edges, and the patient's predisposition to hypertrophic scars.[1,8,10,17]

There are several techniques for hairline correction (**Fig. 2A–C**). Each method has its advantages and disadvantages. Some FFS teams offer techniques for one-stage hair transplantation from excised flaps. Other techniques of hairline correction include hair transplantation simultaneous with forehead reconstruction. There exist different opinions on the timing of hair transplantation, with some groups recommending immediate transplantation and others suggesting that delayed hair transplantation improves engraftment rates and results in fewer complications. Although some argue that hair transplantation is superior to hairline lowering surgery, a consensus has not been reached yet.

Hairline advancement reduces the length of the nonhair-bearing forehead through a pretrichial coronal incision extending posteriorly in the temporal area of the scalp and inferiorly down to the postauricular area. The dissection proceeds posteriorly in either the subgaleal or subperiosteal plane to the occiput to maximally advance the scalp. Galeotomies and intraoperative tissue expansion, checkerboard incisions to loosen the galea can be used for further advancement, although care must be taken to preserve the scalp vascular plexus in the subcutaneous connective tissue layer. Care must be taken to avoid injury to the frontal branch of the facial nerve lying superficial to the deep temporal fascia during the dissection above the temporal bone of the scalp.[13,14,16]

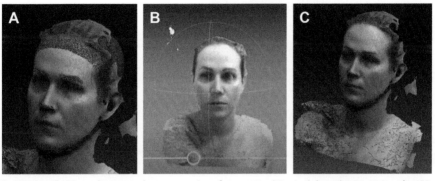

Fig. 1. (*A–C*) 3D - photography apps using for create 3D-model and export to the 3D-modeling tools.

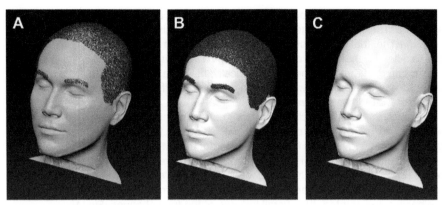

Fig. 2. (A–C) Several techniques for hairline correction.

Forehead reconstruction and adaptation of the hairline always result in some hair follicles being removed. While it is tempting to harvest these follicles and use them for further hair transplantation, practice shows that the survival of these grafts is low. For maximum uptake of grafts, there must be the following conditions: minimal edema in the intervention area (general corticosteroid injections are used to correct

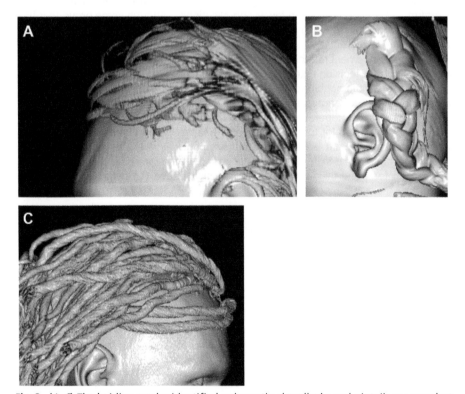

Fig. 3. (A–C) The hairline can be identified only partly, dreadlocks and pigtails are seen but create confusion for the program and the hairline area is never visualized in Tomography.

this condition), the absence of a pressure bandage, and sleeping in a semi-sitting position. However, these conditions contradict the circumstances arising after forehead reconstruction. Accordingly, the number of established grafts during one-stage transplantation and forehead reconstruction will be less.

Correcting the hairline through hairline lowering, it is possible to apply a zigzag scar technique. The advantage of a zigzag incision for correcting the hairline is a more natural hairline shape. It should also be noted that after moving the hairline, hair growth on hormone therapy continues, and sometimes new vellus hairs grow that partially cover the scar. However, the method has some disadvantages. First, the length of the incision increases several times, which implies more bleeding from the area of the vessels of the scalp. There are also some difficulties with the matching of the wound edges, (which can be partially solved by using premodeled templates).

Hairline advancement and frontal bone reduction are generally performed simultaneously, although both procedures have significant variations according to the surgeon's preference. In the process of altering the frontal bone, the orbit also changes to achieve a more feminine appearance. Hairline correction is possible both simultaneously with the correction of the frontal bone and as an independent surgical treatment.

All the patients we operate on undergo multi-spiral computer tomography in the preoperative period. With the use of DICOM viewer, the images are segmented, and 3d meshes of face and skull are created. The mesh is opened in a program for 3d sculpting (we prefer to use "Z-brush" - digital sculpting tool for sculpting and painting), which used for accurate planning of the FFS operations. It is possible to plan hairline transition, and exact millimeters of hairline movement with this method. Additionally, stencils for osteotomies can be created and it also gives an opportunity to understand the needed volume of augmentation of some face areas if facial implants or fat grafts are needed. From this program, the hairline can be identified only partly, dreadlocks and pigtails are seen but create confusion for the program and the hairline area is never visualized in Tomography. Anthropometric measurements, photos, or 3d surface scans (even from mobile) can be used to identify hair projection for defining the hairline. When analyzing the hairline, we emphasize the importance of the balance of the height of chin and hairline, and this can be modeled in 3d planning.[6,12] As the goal is, the smaller the height of the chin, the lower the hairline (**Fig. 3**).

SUMMARY

Hairline lowering and shaping of the silhouette characteristic of women play a great role in facial feminization surgery. The upper third of the face and hairline area is an important factor in gender identification by observers.[2,9,11] Today, among the methods of hairline correction, we cannot choose the ideal method of surgical treatment. Each method must be discussed and agreed upon with the patient. The methods vary widely in cost, pain level, and the duration of the rehabilitation period. It is worthwhile to follow a certain concept in hairline surgery; but the design of the new growth line must be also discussed with the patient. 3D modeling allows you to visually demonstrate the changes that await the patient after the surgery, and come to an accurate understanding of the patient's expectations and the realistic possibilities of the operation.

REFERENCES

1. Capitán L, Simon D, Meyer T, et al. Facial feminization surgery: simultaneous hair transplant during forehead reconstruction. Plast Reconstr Surg 2017;139(3): 573–84.

2. Pansritum K. Forehead and hairline surgery for gender affirmation. Plast Reconstr Surg Glob Open 2021;9(3):e3486.
3. Capitán L, Simon D, Bailón C, et al. The upper third in facial gender confirmation surgery. J Craniofac Surg 2019;30(5):1393–8.
4. Campanella S, Chrysochoos A, Bruyer R. Categorical perception of facial gender information: behavioural evidence and the face-space metaphor. Vis Cogn 2001; 8(2):237–62.
5. Morrison SD, Vyas KS, Motakef S, et al. Facial feminization. Plast Reconstr Surg 2016;137(6):1759–70.
6. Mandelbaum M, Lakhiani C, Chao JW. A novel application of virtual surgical planning to facial feminization surgery. J Craniofac Surg 2019;30(5):1347–8.
7. Jain A, Huang J, Shiaofen F. Gender identification using frontal facial images. IEEE Int Conf Multimedia Expo 2005. https://doi.org/10.1109/icme.2005.1521613.
8. Ousterhout DK. Feminization of the forehead: contour changing to improve female aesthetics. Plast Reconstr Surg 1987;79:701–13.
9. Dang BN, Hu AC, Bertrand AA, et al. Evaluation and treatment of facial feminization surgery: part I. forehead, orbits, eyebrows, eyes, and nose. Arch Plast Surg 2021;48(5):503–10.
10. Neidel FG, Leonhardt K, Finner AM. Hair transplantation in women and transgender patients—general rules and a case report. Hair Transpl Forum Int 2017; 27(6):221–7.
11. Altman K. Facial feminization surgery: current state of the art. Int J Oral Maxillofac Surg 2012;41(8):885–94. https://doi.org/10.1016/j.ijom.2012.04.024.
12. Toma A, Zhurov A, Playle R, et al. A three-dimensional look for facial differences between males and females in a British-Caucasian sample aged 15years old. Orthod Craniofac Res 2008;11(3):180–5. https://doi.org/10.1111/j.1601-6343.2008.00428.x.
13. Shapiro R, Shapiro P. Hairline design and frontal hairline restoration. Facial Plast Surg Clin North Am 2013;21(3):351–62.
14. Unger RH. Female hair restoration. Facial Plast Surg Clin North Am 2013;21(3): 407–17.
15. Bachelet JT, Souchere B, Mojallal A, et al. Facial feminization surgery—upper third. Ann Chir Plast Esthet 2016;61:877–81.
16. Cho SW, Jin HR. Feminization of the forehead in a transgender: frontal sinus reshaping combined with brow lift and hairline lowering. Aesthetic Plast Surg 2012; 36:1207–10.
17. Ainsworth TA, Spiegel JH. Quality of life of individuals with and without facial feminization surgery or gender reassignment surgery. Qual Life Res 2010;19: 1019–24. https://doi.org/10.1007/s11136-010-9668-7.

FURTHER READING

Rodman R, et al. Hairline restoration: difference in men and woman—length and shape. Facial Plast Surg 2018;34(2):155–8. https://doi.org/10.1055/s-0038-1636905.

Moving?

Make sure your subscription moves with you!

To notify us of your new address, find your **Clinics Account Number** (located on your mailing label above your name), and contact customer service at:

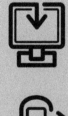

Email: journalscustomerservice-usa@elsevier.com

800-654-2452 (subscribers in the U.S. & Canada)
314-447-8871 (subscribers outside of the U.S. & Canada)

Fax number: 314-447-8029

Elsevier Health Sciences Division
Subscription Customer Service
3251 Riverport Lane
Maryland Heights, MO 63043

*To ensure uninterrupted delivery of your subscription, please notify us at least 4 weeks in advance of move.

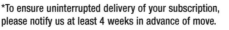